1989

HUMAN LIFE AND MEDICAL PRACTICE

Human Life
and
Medical Practice

J. K. MASON

Regius Professor (Emeritus) of Forensic Medicine
University of Edinburgh

EDINBURGH UNIVERSITY PRESS

© J. K. Mason 1988
Edinburgh University Press
22 George Square, Edinburgh

Set in Linoterm Goudy by
Speedspools, Edinburgh, and
printed in Great Britain by
Redwood Burn Limited
Trowbridge, Wilts.

British Library Cataloguing
  in Publication Data
Mason J. K. (John Kenyon), 1919-
Human life and medical practice.
1. Medicine. Ethical aspects
I. Title
174'.2
ISBN 0 85224 560 2
ISBN 0 85224 584 x Pbk

Contents

v

This book is dedicated to my sons
IAN and PAUL.
who disagree with most of what I say

All men do not reflect truly and accurately, so as to do justice to their own meanings; but only in proportion to their abilities and attainments. In other words, all men have a reason, but not all men can give a reason.

John (later Cardinal) Newman, 1843

Preface

It is nearly half a century since I qualified in medicine and it needs no preface to describe the vast changes which have come about during that period in the diagnosis, prevention and treatment of disease. Medical practice has become scientifically based and offers the patient an expertise that would have been regarded as science fiction before the Second World War. At the same time, while doctors' work has become more time-consuming and stressful, patients have become more demanding and it would be idle to deny that the doctor/patient relationship has become relatively impersonal—at least, in the hospital environment.

A further inevitable result of the modern, scientific approach to medicine is that it leads to a quest for human perfection and that, along the road to that goal, those who are irrevocably imperfect tend to get left behind—this includes the congenitally deformed, the neonate and the terminally ill. Attitudes to the value of life must change and it is well to stand back occasionally to see where we are going.

I admit to being concerned that we are becoming too ready to devalue the imperfect and, for that reason, I have wanted to write this book for some time. But it must be regarded as no more than a cautionary review; it may, at times, appear critical but that is not its primary intention. No one is more conscious than I am of the devotion which goes into caring for the newborn, for the paralysed or for the patient with disseminated cancer; what one would hope is that the whole profession would be motivated by the ideals of these specialists. This book will have served its purpose if it indicates ways or means by which this could come about.

The subjects covered are very emotional and must inevitably be subjectively coloured. It is important that authors in this field show their colours and I think it only fair to readers to say that I am a practising Roman Catholic; but this does not mean that I can have no individual conscience. In any case, what I am trying to speak of is the ethical practice of medicine, not the application of religious precept. Any bias in my conclusions is, I hope, attributable to reasonable deduction only.

I owe a debt of gratitude to those who have helped me with temporary typing—in particular, Mrs Liz MacDonald and Mrs Sheila Smith. Dr R. A. McCall Smith has given me valuable criticism of parts of the manuscript. Dr Kenneth Boyd was kind enough to point me to the thematic quotation which exactly matches my feelings of inadequacy in an area which is of profound significance for the law, the public and the medical

profession. Finally, I would like to thank Edinburgh University Press for
their courage and kindness in bringing this slim volume to fruition.

Edinburgh, March 1987   JKM

Introduction

1. A Perspective

The persuasive influence of the ancient Hippocratic Oath was accepted in 1948 when the World Medical Association drew up the Declaration of Geneva. The British Medical Association strongly advocated an international profession of ethical conduct and included in its submission to the WMA:

> The spirit of the Hippocratic Oath cannot change and enjoins the duty of curing, the greatest crime being cooperation in the destruction of life by murder, suicide and abortion. [1]

The emotive tone of this rubric was modified and has survived in the Declaration of Sydney[2]—the 1968 version of the Geneva Declaration — as:

> The health of my patients will be my first consideration . . . I will maintain the utmost respect for human life from the time of conception.

All such declarations are, essentially, compromises in the cause of international agreement and are subject to interpretation and modification at national level. Nevertheless, the Declaration shows that, in 1968, the medical profession was committed to the concept of the sanctity of life—the duty of the doctor was to preserve life and the nature of that duty was unqualified, at least so far as the Declaration of Sydney was concerned.

Yet, in 1973 we read in a paper accepted for publication by the official Journal of the British Medical Association:

> The whole resources of an advanced medical service are currently deployed in the pursuit of the preservation of life . . . We must face an inescapable duty to let some patients die . . . We should regard the prevention of suffering as our primary aim. The preservation of life is secondary and acceptable only if the suffering involved is tolerable and of short term. [3]

Clearly, there had been a marked change of emphasis in only a few years and this philosophy was already being applied on a world-wide basis. Nowhere was this more overt than within the confines of paediatric practice. In England, Lorber had, by 1972, reviewed the results of his treatment of children with neural tube defects and, as a direct consequence of the distressing picture which had evolved, had openly introduced a policy of selective non-treatment. [4] Later, he described the main object of selection as being: 'not to avoid treating those who would die

3

early in spite of treatment but to avoid treating those who would survive with severe handicap'.[5] The same line was being followed in the United States, where it was reported that fourteen per cent of deaths in a special nursery were associated with discontinuance or withdrawal of treatment as a result of decisions made by physicians and parents acting in concert.[6]

The medical profession was clearly moving towards an ethos which was influenced by the concept of preserving the quality of life rather than of endowing life with an absolute value. Moreover, as the quotation from Slater given above indicates, the quality of life was not to be measured only in terms of the individual's status. The idea of the differential allocation of resources—whether on financial, logistic or simply emotional grounds—was being introduced and, with it, account was being taken of the relative quality of the lives of others competing for those resources. All of which indicates a remarkable shift from the Hippocratic position.

Although it is unlikely that any really satisfactory answer will be discovered, it is worth considering whether this transition was so abrupt, or whether the process was as new as is suggested by the wide exposure to which the topic has been subjected in the 1970s and 1980s. Has the shift been the result of an insidious change in the attitudes of society and, particularly, of the medical profession, or have there been violent moral upheavals which have enforced relatively sudden changes in our views on the value of life?

The religious influence

Killing defective or otherwise unwanted newborns or allowing the incapacitated elderly to die by exposure has been accepted in the past as a primitive form of population control. The implication is that man's instinctive reaction in times of stress is to regard the rights of the herd to survival as being greater than those of the non-contributory individual. This instinct was developed into a policy in the great civilisations of the pre-Christian and Roman eras and ranged from the Incas' mass slaughter of sacrifices to protect the community from the wrath of the Gods to the primitive eugenic approach of the Spartans towards their newborn.

The impetus towards the contemporary belief in an individual's absolute right to life derives mainly from the acceptance of monotheistic religion. Whereas it had previously been possible to, so to speak, play one God off against another, the concept of a single creator and single destroyer carried with it an implication of culpability should anyone interfere with His order. God has given life and only God can take it away. Thus, the sanctity of life—the prohibition of procuring or hastening death by any means—is implicit in the Jewish Talmud,[7] in the Koran and in the writings of the early Christian polemicists.[8]

Certain concomitants are implicit in these religious concepts. In the first place, the doctrine that 'God made man in His own image and likeness'—as the Roman Catholic Catechism has it—implies that human life is distinct and carries with it rights and duties which are not shared by the remainder of the animal kingdom. This belief is coming under increasing attack as a manifestation of 'speciesism'.[9] There can be no doubt as to the existence of some animal rights, but to admit to this is not to concede that they are either of the same degree or of the same quality as those of human rights. It matters not whether you adopt the religious concept of ensoulment or the secular appeal to 'personhood'[10] in making a distinction between animal and human life. The distinction is there and it is one which is generally accepted; vegetarianism has never been central to human philosophy, whereas, with few exceptions, human cannibalism has been condemned. In making this distinction there is no intention to decry the motives of those who, say, oppose the wanton killing of animals for pleasure but the issue lies outside the confines of this book; the introduction of the word 'human' into the title is deliberately restrictive.

Secondly, there is a clear implication in the religious view that there should be an absolute duty to preserve all human life on the grounds that all human lives are of equal value in the sight of God. But what of the sight of man? Faced with the immorality of slavery, the moral man must denounce its conditions because they undervalue the humanity of the slave by reducing him to the status of an economic unit. But similar degrading conditions may be dictated by nature rather than by man. The person who is physically disadvantaged may well find life so intolerable that it represents, to him, a nil value and there is then no duty imposed on anyone to maintain a contrary fiction (though the duty to help naturally remains); the doctrine of religious absolutism is thus tempered by that of Kantian autonomy or of self determination. In certain circumstances, this autonomy may have to be expressed in surrogate fashion but this is immaterial to the overall argument. The fact remains that, while religion may not allow persons to take their own lives, the individual is perfectly entitled to apply a value judgment as to the quality of his or her life and to reject treatment or other help in the light of that analysis. The absolute value of human life is, thereby, modified and the greater part of this work is concerned with assessing the impact of this concept on the practice of medicine.

Thirdly, organised religion itself makes exceptions to the absolute sanctity of human life. Thus, many States in which religion has a powerful voice in governmental policy-making retain the judicial death penalty, and the insidious acceptance of war as a legitimate aspect of Christianity and of other faiths has been the subject of frequent comment.[11] Even so, wars, even up to the end of the nineteenth century were, to a large extent, fought on a man to man basis and it was just possible to preserve the sanctity of life principle in part by upholding the fiction that fighting was essentially a matter of self defence.

A changing world

Nevertheless, it was, in my opinion, war—that is the Great War of 1914–18—which provoked the major upheaval in society's attitude to human life. It became impossible to sustain the fundemental religious view of life's value so long as secular leaders were willing and empowered to destroy thousands of men in a single day and in a wholly anonymous fashion. Such rejectionist leanings were reinforced a generation later by the barbarities exemplified by the razing of Coventry, Dresden and Nagasaki or by the almost equally impersonal atrocities of Auschwitz or the Burma Road. Whether it be a matter of *propter hoc* or *post hoc*, society coincidentally began to turn against organised religion as an arbiter of national policy. The immediate effect of that movement was to have a particularly profound effect in the current context insofar as religious conviction is the main buttress of the sanctity of life ethos. In its place, a massive groundswell arose towards self determination and towards the right to the disposal of one's own person—effectively a return to the philosophy of J. S. Mill:

> The only purpose for which power can rightfully be exercised over any member of a civilised community against his will is to prevent harm to others . . . He cannot rightfully be compelled to do or forebear because it would be better for him to do so, because it would make him happy or because, in the opinion of others, to do so would be wise, or even right. [12]

The major thrust of private law since the Second World War has been directed along these libertarian lines. The first significant breakthrough in the context of the 'life debate' came with the passing of the Suicide Act 1961. The particular moral significance of this lay in the contrast now made apparent between the new secular legislation and the still unaltered condemnation of self killing by all monotheistic religions; religion and law were parting company in a pluralistic, and largely agnostic, society.

The Suicide Act had very little direct effect on the medical profession other than to clarify the fact that non-consensual treatment of the would-be suicide was wrongful. However, the distinction between suicide and voluntary euthanasia—which will be discussed in greater detail later—is not great. The indirect effect of the Act, and of the debate leading up to its passage, was, therefore, to focus attention on the many decisions which need to be made at the interface of life and death and in which the medical profession must play a major role. But, while the profession's innate paternalism and seclusion was sufficient to deflect public review and criticism of doctors' standards for some time, the increasing influence of 'rights movements'—particularly in the field of patients' rights—has led to a profound recent change in attitudes and to increasing demands for public accountability of doctors. [13]

I have argued elsewhere[14] that none of the accepted basic theories of philosophy covers the full range of medical ethics entirely satisfactorily. The ethical practice of medicine rests on an uneasy confederation of deontology, religion, utilitarianism and self determination and, being a public service, its pattern is ultimately shaped by the public conscience. It is, therefore, possible to argue[15] that any professional shift from a sanctity of life to a quality of life position has been no more than a reflection of trends in the social ambience and that the widely publicised conceptual upheavals as to patient management over the 1970s and 1980s do not indicate a particular deviation on the part of medical practitioners. The apparent changes derive mainly from the rapid technological advances in medicine – which are of such extent that it is now fair to say that a natural death is a rarity.[16] The great majority of deaths in the United Kingdom now occur in hospital where all modern techniques can be applied. It is not, say the apologists, the decisions which have changed but, rather, the environment in which they are made. If that environment is subject to increasing publicity—both intrusive of and self-seeking by the profession—then the public's appetite for matters medical is merely being properly satisfied.

A time is likely to come, however, when the relatively gentle tempo of subscription to external changes is disrupted—a time when the medical profession has to stand and make an assessment of its position in relation to the public. Such a situation was presented in classic form with the passing of the Abortion Act 1967—an Act which effectively eliminated a major Hippocratic principle of the medical profession. The Act was so drafted that the saving of a mother's life—which is the only indication for abortion which is still compatible with a sanctity of life ethos[17]—became a numerically insignificant reason for a therapeutic operation.

The central issue of abortion will be considered in detail in a later chapter. As one who was practising in the early 1960s, I can testify to the strength of conservative resistance to the Act to be found within the rank and file of the profession. For present purposes, however, the outstanding feature of the abortion controversy is that the medical establishment—and particularly the British Medical Association—accepted and, indeed, embraced the policy enforced by the legislature. 'Doctors take the view [that there is no need for any amendment to the Act] because they know that in general the Act is working well'.[18]

This can only be seen as a watershed in medical ethics from which there is, effectively, no return. Whether or not it is possible to argue that abortion does not involve the taking of 'life' will be discussed later. The fact remains that its immediate and unquestioned acceptance by the profession's political leaders involved a simultaneous revocation of a previously deeply held conviction. If such a change is possible in respect of one Hippocratic imperative, there is no compelling reason why it should not be repeated in other tenets, for example: 'I will follow that system or regimen which, according to my ability and judgment, I consider for the benefit of my patient and abstain from whatever is deleterious and mischievous'. Whether we like it or not, the profession's reaction to the Abortion Act must colour any discussion of its current ethics in relation to the value of life.

The problems posed

But what if the law is unclear—as it may well be in the absence of statute or legal precedent? What if doctors, having once abrogated a fundamental principle, choose to enter, or are forced into, uncharted waters? The publication of articles under such headings as, on the one hand, 'The legal threat to medicine'[19] and, on the other, 'Doctors as murderers'[20] indicates the potential for conflict. This is an unhappy situation. 'Society' said Beynon 'can afford the luxury of this sort of dissension, indecision and delay. Doctors and their patients cannot'.

The issues are of immediate practical significance. Dunn, giving evidence at the trial of Dr Arthur (discussed in detail later) is reported as saying: 'No paediatrician takes life but we accept that allowing babies to die is in the baby's interest at times'[21]—and he was widely supported in giving such testimony. This statement embodies a number of assumptions:

(a) that there is an essential difference between activity and passivity when the same end—death—can be realised by either and, arising from this:

   (i) that passivity does not conflict with our duty to 'maintain the utmost respect for human life'.
   (ii) that passivity is clinically preferable—that is, preferable from the point of view of the patient.

(b) that there is a point at which death is preferable to life and that this is agreed in medical, legal and public circles.

(c) that someone can *make* that decision in surrogate fashion and

(d) that it is right and proper for some person to act on that assumption.

Yet there is no certainty that any such implications are true in law nor, even, that the principles are acceptable to the majority of society or of the medical profession. The purpose of this book is, therefore, to examine the current medico-legal situation in respect of the medical profession's attitude to life and to make recommendations for the future. The abortion issue is now settled—the Act is with us and is here to stay. Nevertheless, the issues raised by abortion are fundamental to the whole discussion of life and death decisions. Moreover, they have recently resurfaced within the context of the *in vitro* fertilisation programme. Elsewhere, right to life or right to death decisions must be taken without specific statutory guidance at several points in life and each of these points poses its own particular problems. I therefore, propose to discuss the issues at four levels—at the end of life's span, during adulthood, in the immediately post-natal period and before birth.

Life and Death Decisions

2. Terminal Illness

In view of the importance attached to abortion, it may seem paradoxical to begin a discussion of life and death decisions at the end of life. The rationale for this is that, on the face of things, it is at this time that there ought to be least difficulty—both clinically and morally—in therapeutic decision-making. By definition, terminal implies that there is minimal potential for a future life of any quality. This is the classic situation in which we *know* that we are doing no more than prolonging the process of dying;[1] treatment, even if successful, can be described as such for only the shortest possible time.

It is important to be clear that this is a condition which is strictly confined. Failure in this respect leads to a confusion of aims and principles.[2] Thus, in the Incurable Patients Bill 1976—which failed by a substantial majority in the House of Lords—the 'incurable patient' was defined as one who is: 'suffering without any reasonable prospect of cure from a distressing physical illness or disability that he finds intolerable'. The clause thus widened the scope of the debate to include not only the terminally ill but also, say, sufferers from rheumatoid arthritis. This represents a considerable retreat from a sanctity of life principle, and it is interesting to note how deeply entrenched that principle was in the minds of our more enlightened legislators at that time.[3]

Although the subject has not since been raised in Parliament, the concept of incurable disease has continued to widen significantly over the years in medical, legal and philosophical circles. This movement has increasingly tended to correlate the value of life with what McCormick defined many years ago as 'the potentiality for human relationships':[4] attention is thereby concentrated on cerebral function. The idea that the intrinsic quality of life is defined by the ability of the brain to support the body, originally posed in the context of artificial life support,[5] inexorably leads to a questioning of the value of those persons who are so affected mentally as to be unable to look after themselves—'may not *homo sapiens* be weakened if he devotes resources to *homo* who is no longer *sapiens*?'[6]—and, before long, termination of life is listed as a credible option in the management of diseases of the central nervous system which are specific to old age.[7]

Euthanasia has generally been taken to describe an easy death or death without suffering but *Collins English Dictionary*, for example, defines it as: 'the act of killing someone painlessly'—and it is in this rather more

13

pejorative sense that the term is now more commonly used. To confuse the two separate issues—terminal and incurable illness—is to fail to distinguish between care of the dying and 'euthanasia'—this being a point which was taken up in the debate on the 1976 Bill. For the present, therefore, discussion is limited to decisions which are to be taken within the confines of terminal illness.

Definitive treatment

The ethical issues surrounding the treatment of conscious but terminally ill patients are now largely settled both medically and legally speaking. The dying patient is as autonomous as is the young adult; treatment of any sort is subject to his or her consent and the rules relating to consent are similar irrespective of life expectancy.

A digression into a full discussion on the nature of consent[8] would be out of place here; nevertheless, there are some aspects of the doctrine which are particularly apposite to the conditions of terminal care and a brief explanation related to that task will not be out of place. Broadly speaking, consent to a specific form of treatment is based on what is generally known as 'informed consent'. This term was imported from the United States and, although it is widely used, it is of doubtful validity in the United Kingdom following Dunn LJ's comment that: 'the doctrine of informed consent forms no part of English law'.[9] One suspects that the statement may contain an element of semantic misinterpretation but it is, nevertheless, simpler and more consistent to speak now in terms of rational consent. To do so also underlines the basic principle of the doctrine which is that the patient has a right to make a rational decision as to acceptance or refusal of treatment based on his understanding of the information which the doctor gives him. The amount of information to be given is governed by medical practice which is accepted at the time as proper by a responsible body of medical opinion—subject, as always, to the right of the Court to decide on the definition of 'proper'.[10] Two more definitive criteria can be elicited from recent litigation. Firstly, while the doctor is under no obligation to prompt questioning, he must answer such questions as are put to him truthfully and honestly; secondly, and of particular interest in the context of the terminally ill, he is entitled to what is known as 'therapeutic privilege'—that is to say, he may withhold information which he thinks may be deleterious to the well-being of his patient.

The provision of information is regarded as being part of the general treatment of the patient—something which may be very difficult in these particular circumstances and which will depend, to a large extent, not only on the mental state of the patient but also on the maintenance of a 'therapeutic alliance' in particularly distressing conditions. It follows that a doctor's failure to convey information adequately, thus hindering the patient from making a rational decision, may be regarded as negligence and, therefore, as being actionable in tort; the corollary is that a general consent to treatment, as opposed to consent to a specific procedure, elides a potential trespass to the person. An action in battery exists, however, if no consent is obtained or if consent is obtained by fraud or misrepresentation; treatment against the patient's express wishes would certainly be regarded as a trespass and could, conceivably, have criminal implications. [11] Thus, the doctor not only has no mandate to continue treatment against the patient's wishes but, in so doing, he is also possibly guilty of professional misconduct. It was, therefore, rightly said in the debate on the Incurable Patients Bill 1976 that there was no legal need for legislation allowing a patient to refuse treatment; he already has that right even if exercising it is likely to result in accelerated death.

It must be noted, however, that this common law right is subject to qualification. The conditions under which the State may legitimately intervene have been emphasised particularly in the United States where they can be summarised under four headings: (a) a general interest in the preservation of life both of the individual and of the sanctity of all life; (b) the need to protect innocent third parties; (c) the duty to prevent suicide; and (d) an interest in safeguarding the integrity of the medical profession. [12] All these exceptions have a potential effect on the sanctity of life debate and all are raised, directly or indirectly, in parts of this book. In the present context, it is the all-embracing interest in the preservation of life which has major significance but, so long as the particular life involved is that of the decision-maker, the State's interest generally gives way to the patient's much stronger personal interest in directing the course of his own life: 'Governmental tolerance of the choice to resist treatment reflects concern for individual self-determination, bodily integrity, and avoidance of suffering, rather than a depreciation of life's value'. [13] The position in the United Kingdom, while not being codified to the same extent, is very similar; directions as to the management of hunger-strikers indicate the importance attached to personal autonomy even in the face of possibly serious political repercussions. [14]

By contrast, it may be asked if the patient has any absolute entitlement to treatment on demand? Everyone has a claim to cling to life if they can do so without detriment to others. In this connection, the medical problems associated with the allocation of scarce therapeutic resources are very real although they are best discussed in the more practical context of intensive care (see below). But what if the terminally ill patient calls for treatment which the doctor knows will be, at best, ineffective and, at worst, mutilating or even lethal, but which yet lies within his competence? It is clear that, in law, a doctor does not have to save life merely by reason of his qualifications; he does not have to perform an operation he does not want to perform and, in the event of the patient's death, he would not be guilty of homicide by failing to do so. [15] If this is so when life can be salvaged, it must be doubly so in the face of terminal illness and the doctor would be fully entitled, after due explanation, to refuse a case in which he considered treatment would be improper and, if necessary, to refer the patient to a colleague. This might, however, be difficult in the hospital environment. Moreover, terminal medical care involves treatment of the whole person and, to that extent, to refuse the patient's wishes is to deny him such a minimum quality of life as is available and is of his own choosing. The situation envisaged is unusual and one on which it is difficult to generalise. It is submitted, however, that it would be not only morally but also logically right in such a case to operate the doctrine of 'rational consent', so to speak, in reverse; the futility of the procedure, its dangers and its possible side effects having been explained, the doctor should, whenever feasible, bow to the wishes of the autonomous patient. So long as this was the clear line of intent, no opprobrium would fall on the doctor for the inevitable failure—he would be further immune from criticism because, within the National Health Service, there would be no financial overtones which might otherwise be implied from his keeping the patient alive to no purpose.

The National Health Service structure, however, does not always operate to simplify physicians' problems, insofar as economic considerations tend to be obscured within a service in which the consumer, or patient, is absolved from financial constraints. Resources within that service must all be finite and the doctor cannot exclude their distribution from his response to patients' requests. Once again, it is only possible to say, perhaps tritely, that the individual case can only be decided on its particular merits at that particular time. To what extent does the individual's wish justify the consumption of resources—be they of manpower, finance, bed space or actual materials? How far will others be immediately affected by what appears to be an inappropriate use? There can be no overall positive reply to such questions—the best that evolves from discussion of the issue is that allocation decisions must be made on moral grounds and not by arbitrary methods, including partiality; [16] at all events, beneficence, or doing good, must take precedence over benevolence or do-gooding. Negatively, however, it is surely right to say that a resource, no matter how allocated, cannot be withdrawn later simply because a more deserving candidate appears. The importance of making the decision to *admit* a patient to a resource of whatever nature cannot be over-emphasised and the matter is discussed in greater detail in relation to intensive care (p.46).

Despite the foregoing, the situation of the fully competent but dying patient which more commonly needs to be considered is summed up in the opposing question—what should be the doctor's attitude as to the sanctity of life if the patient positively requests death? In my experience, the problem arises far less often than might be supposed. When faced with death, the vast majority of patients will hold on to life with determination, and this is particularly so when they are supported by a loving family or by the services of a modern hospice. The request, when made, is not so much 'relieve me of my life' as 'relieve me of my pain'. This latter, and major, therapeutic objective lies at the heart of the modern Hippocratic conscience and its ethical basis must be considered in detail.

The relief of pain

The field of discussion must now be extended. There can, of course, be no doubt over the legal fact that murder is murder irrespective of the state of the victim:

> If the acts done are intended to kill and do, in fact, kill, it does not matter if the life of the victim is shortened by months or weeks, or even hours or minutes, it is still murder. [17]

Nevertheless, there is an emotional and practical distinction between drawing the final curtain on the last scene of life—which is a natural part of the scenario—and interrupting the play even before the last act is reached, which is not. Any discussion on the termination of life, by whatever means, must include pre-terminal conditions if it is to be intelligible and, to that extent, we are now shifting our ground.

The doctor's therapeutic function has two facets. First, he can treat disease. If he gives an appropriate antibiotic in a case of bacterial infection, he is striking at a fundamental cause of ill health and, in general, nothing but good can come of his action. All too often, however, this course is closed to him—either because there is no basic treatment or because the condition results from irreparable degeneration or destruction of tissue. In these circumstances, his secondary purpose is to treat symptoms, and the most urgent of these is pain.

Discussion of the interplay between analgesia and accelerated death is, to some extent, being outmoded by the quality of treatment practised within the modern hospice movement. Used in this environment, pain-killing drugs such as morphine are thought to have little adverse effect on life expectancy. [18] In normal practice, however, it is to be anticipated that increasing doses of narcotic analgesics will endanger life; and while it is reasonable to regard this as reflecting bad medical practice, it is the outcome which will be accepted as probable in the commentary which follows.

The moral position

The concept of relieving pain at the expense of shortening life epitomises the conflict between the quality and sanctity of life doctrines. Following the general retreat from the latter, there are now very few doctors whose inclinations would not be to give priority to the relief of symptoms when the choice is demanded; the practice must, however, be justified both morally and legally.

The moral solution is reasonably clear and is based on the doctrine of 'double effect'. Simplistically, this holds that so long as there is no less injurious alternative, an action is permissible when its intended good effect can only be obtained at the expense of, and in the expectation of, a coincidental ill-effect. The full doctrine is, however, subject to certain pre-requisites: the action itself must be either good or morally indifferent, the good effect must not be produced by means of the ill-effect and there must be a proportionate reason for allowing the expected ill to occur.[19] The principle is widely accepted in Christian theology, the Roman Catholic authority being Pope Pius XII who replied 'Yes—if no other means exist' to the prepared question: 'Is the suppression of pain and consciousness by the use of narcotics . . . permitted by religion and morality to the doctor and the patient even . . . if one foresees that the use of narcotics will shorten life?'[20] This precept has been reaffirmed, although with slight modifications allowing for the Christian virtue of suffering.[21] The general agreement of the Church of England was reiterated by the Archbishop of Canterbury in 1977.[22] In this paper, he quoted the Anglican canon lawyer, E. G. Moore, as saying:

> It would seem reasonably certain that the giving of a pain killing drug to a patient in extremis can be justified not only by the theologian's law of double effect but also by the common law doctrine of necessity even where one of the effects of the drug is the probable shortening of the patient's life.[23]

The doctor's ethical position is, thus, settled but, at the same time, it must be appreciated that the application of the 'double effect' doctrine involves a value judgment, the foundations for which may vary. It may be perfectly clear that the life expectancy of an already moribund patient is a minor factor in therapeutic decision-making; it is far less clear that a young person in similar pain, but with a prognosis which allows scope for the introduction of new treatments, should be put at similar risk—the balance of good/evil, or the proportionate reason in this case has shifted significantly. Ultimately, such problems can only be resolved on the basis of good clinical judgment. But that judgment inevitably erodes the sancity of life principle—a pain-free death is preferred to a painful life.

The legal position

The legal counterpart of the 'double effect' doctrine is that of necessity which applies the principle that acting unlawfully is justified if the resulting good materially outweighs the consequences of adhering strictly to the law. The immediate relevance of the principle to medical treatment is not, however, entirely straightforward. Professor Glanville Williams, in fact, made much of a *distinction* between double effect and necessity. In 1958, he wrote as to the former:

There is no legal difference between desiring or intending a consequence as following from your conduct, and persisting in your
conduct with a knowledge that the consequence will inevitably
follow from it, though not desiring that consequence. When a
result is foreseen as certain, it is the same as if it were desired or
intended.[24]

At the same time, however, he was fully prepared to accept necessity
as absolving the doctor from blame:

The fact is that there is no logical or moral chasm between what
may be called shortening life and accelerating death. Once admit
the principle that a physician may knowingly, for sufficient reason,
shorten a patient's expectation of life . . . and one is compelled to
admit that he may knowingly, for sufficient reason, put an end to his
patient's life immediately . . . this line of argument tends to show
that a physician may give any amount of drug necessary to deaden
pain, even though he knows that that amount will bring about
speedy or indeed immediate death. His legal excuse does not rest
upon the Roman Church's doctrine of 'double effect' . . . the excuse
rests upon the doctrine of necessity.[25]

The distinction is not easy to appreciate and, indeed, much of the
chapter, written by a great lawyer, reads somewhat strangely to a non-
lawyer because of its concern to distinguish the doctor as being, in some
ways, apart from others who might feel equally attracted by the 'merciful
release' theory. Nevertheless, Williams is confident of the application of
the necessity doctrine to the treatment of terminal illness[26] and many
American lawyers would agree.[27]

There are, however, other contrary expressions of view. We find Lord
Edmund-Davies saying in 1977:

Doing nothing or killing both the pain and the patient who has only
a short life to live . . . may be good morals but it is far from clear that
it is good law[28]

and quoting Lord Hailsham LC:

The law at the moment is perfectly plain: if you have got a living
body, you have to keep it alive, if you can.[29]

In the face of such conflicting of views, one must look to the precedent
of case law but here again the material is scanty and not entirely
convincing. The only truly apposite case is *R v Adams*.[30]

Dr Adams' patient was not dying when she was treated with increasing
amounts of narcotic drugs which were thought to have killed her. The
doctor was charged with murder and was acquitted by the jury; Devlin J's
summing up has been very widely quoted, and his comments on the law
of murder have already been noted.[17] Elsewhere, however, he said:

The doctor . . . is entitled to do all that is proper and necessary to
relieve pain and suffering even if the measures he takes may incidentally shorten life.

The case of Dr Adams is not easy. It is widely thought to illustrate the importance in the criminal courts of the defence of necessity in therapeutic killing. Williams, however,[31] saw, with some regret, the judge's charge to the jury as conceding the possibility of a defence under the legal theory of causation. 'No act is murder which does not cause death', said Devlin J; the conclusion drawn by Williams is that, although death may legally be preferred to great pain, it probably may not, under the existing law, be preferred to existence in a state of drugged torpor.

It may, therefore, be asked whether *Adams* has the significance for the medical profession and, hence, for the profession's right to therapeutic privilege which has been claimed. In an article which was strongly critical of legal intervention in medicine,[32] the Secretary of the British Medical Association upbraided the Director of Public Prosecutions for saying: 'Doctors who deliberately speed death could face the prospect of life imprisonment'. Havard followed up his criticism by stating that, if the direction in *Adams* was to be overturned, then he, for one, was going to make sure he died out of England.[33] The reason for this fear is not immediately apparent. The major thrust of the *Adams* direction was to distinguish between intent and motive. The DPP's use of the word 'deliberately' was, I suspect, fully calculated and his statement accurately expresses not only the state of the law but of the law as most doctors understand it. Whether or not *Adams* is a true precedent, there seems no reason to suppose that, *pace* Lord Edmund-Davies, a defence of necessity would be denied a doctor who honestly believed he was acting in the best interests of his patient.

This brings us to the second conclusion to be drawn from the case—that, in general, juries will be very reluctant to convict a doctor in such circumstances. They may, as Williams indicated, acquit even when the evidence and the judge's direction leaves them with no legal reason for doing so. They are certainly very unlikely to convict a doctor of murder so long as the crime carries a mandatory sentence of life imprisonment.

This leads to a third question rather than conclusion—is this an ideal situation? The distinction between affecting life expectancy—which, according to Devlin J, does not constitute murder, and causing death—which does—is a fine one and every profession has its sinners as well as its saints. Dr Adams had, admittedly, falsified his patient's cremation certificate and there were undercurrents of his having a pecuniary interest in her death. Following Dr Adams' death, Devlin J took the unusual step of publishing his reflections on the trial[34] and he is now far from convinced that acquittal was just. It will be argued later, in the context of the newborn, that the true public reaction to therapeutic killing, as expressed in the law, is unlikely to be discovered until the emotions of the jury are calmed by being required to judge a trial on a lesser charge than one of murder or attempted murder. In the event of a second Dr Adams, an indictment for manslaughter would, perhaps, evoke a more useful indication of how society sees the doctor's role in preserving life. The alternative is, of course, to change the law. Lord Edmund-Davies[35] has suggested that a doctor might:

Prefer to proceed within the known protection of the law rather than be left to act in the hope that those charged with law enforcement would turn a blind eye to what in mercy [he] felt compelled to do . . .

and, in some circumstances to be discussed later, this may well be so.

Williams[36] has suggested a formula based on the Infant Life (Preservation) Act 1929 which would provide that:

No medical practitioner should be guilty in respect of an act done intentionally to accelerate the death of a patient who is seriously ill, unless it is proved that the act was not done in good faith with the consent of the patient and for the purpose of saving him from severe pain in an illness believed to be of an untreatable and fatal character.

Such a measure would be both enabling yet, at the same time, limiting—judging by previous experience, and despite the very great advantages of clarity, it would be likely to be rejected by the medical establishment on the latter ground.[37] Whether or not it would seriously affect the existing state of the law, it would go some way to codifying it and, as such, there is much to commend the suggestion. Williams' formula, however, goes further than to regularise the treatment of terminal illness. It intentionally opens the way to legal euthanasia, controversy over which has been, and remains, intense.

3. Euthanasia

Once euthanasia is defined in terms such as painless killing, the boundaries of the sanctity/quality of life debate are greatly extended. Discussion is no longer confined to such sophisticated niceties as the pharmacological dose of morphine; the intention in euthanasia is the death of the patient. Moreover, the subject embraces a broad spectrum of disease, much of which may have no intrinsic fatal component. Just as the manic depressive may find his life intolerable and often seeks to make an end to it, so may the life of the demented arteriosclerotic seem valueless to others who may, then, feel constrained to bring it to a rapid close. Euthanasia is unconfined by age limits. It is true that much of the discussion inevitably centres on the senescent but the principles of euthanasia may be applied to the middle aged arthritic, to the young adult who is injured or to the infant with congenital defects. These age groups all have their particular problems but it is appropriate, here, to confine discussion to general principles.

Euthanasia is generally considered as being practised in active or in passive form. Each of these is regarded as being either voluntary or involuntary in nature. Glover[1] adds a further 'non-voluntary' category which covers those instances when 'the patient is either not in a position to have, or is not in a position to express, any views on the matter [of his life or death]'. Non-voluntary euthanasia thus includes ending the lives of neonates and of the comatose, each of which presents such specific problems as to merit distinct consideration (chapters 5 and 6). The mentally handicapped, in particular the senile demented, are less certainly distinguished and their management is discussed later in this section.

There then remain four classic types of euthanasia. Two of these—voluntary passive and voluntary active—dictate the co-operation of the patient by definition. The former does no more than express the autonomous right of the patient to refuse treatment; as such, it is a theme which recurs constantly throughout this book. The latter is conceptually, if not legally, so closely allied to suicide as to be better considered under that heading (chapter 4). By contrast, involuntary euthanasia, whether active or passive, excludes the patient from decision-making. Other parties, such as relatives, may be concerned as participants but, in the greater part, involuntary euthanasia will be an expression of medical paternalism: it is the doctor who assesses the quality of the patient's life and it is the doctor who decides whether or not it should be preserved. It is this aspect of euthanasia which forms the main body of this chapter— although the same principles can, obviously, be followed in the non-voluntary situation.

Passive involuntary euthanasia

There is much to be said for abandoning the term 'passive involuntary euthanasia' in favour of 'selective non-treatment'. The latter term describes exactly what is involved. It also has the merit of expressing a major conceptual difference between active and passive processes— selective non-treatment will only result in the death of the patient if there is a treatable condition which will be fatal in the absence of appropriate therapy. This limitation, as has been pointed out already, does not apply to the active termination of life. Nevertheless, it is axiomatic that each has the same end in view—the death of the patient; each, therefore, represents an absolute denial of the sanctity of life principle and, since absolutes are of equal value, there is an undoubted case for holding that there is no distinction to be made between passivity and activity in this context. Rachels is, perhaps, the father of this idea[2] which has been taken up recently by the vigorous Australian school of philosophy at Monash University. Kuhse[3] has evolved a telling argument, based on both intention and causation, to show that, insofar as deliberately withholding treatment is a diversion from the normal expectation of the doctor's role, passive involuntary euthanasia is not only morally indistinguishable from active killing but is also, and similarly, murder.

How, then—murder being a serious crime—is the practice of selective non-treatment, which is undoubtedly widely accepted in the medical world, to be justified? One suggestion, which is discussed in greater detail in relation to Arthur (p.70), is that a practice ceases to be reprehensible if enough people adopt it. A custom may, however, evolve for wrong reasons and some moral basis must be demonstrated before it becomes acceptable as part of normal behaviour. For present purposes, there seems to be no alternative but to adopt the utilitarian stance that death from non-treatment is for the ultimate benefit of the patient— which is unsatisfactory in that it fails to explain why active killing should not be equally, or more, beneficial, a point which is reverted to later, particularly in connection with the neonate (chapter 6).

An assessment of benefit involves a value judgment which, in the likely circumstances of selective non-treatment, will be made by the doctor without the patient's knowledge that a choice is being made. There is a suggestion that custom, influenced as it is by the increasing materialism of the modern age, is now operating so as to influence physicians in favour of death when a choice needs to be taken; this may well be a wrong road and one which leads to an underestimation of the

degree to which life, notwithstanding its 'quality', is prized by its owner.
A remarkable study of quadriplegia was published in 1985.[4] A healthy
individual is unlikely to be able to conceive of a worse life-form than to
be paralysed in the arms, legs and trunk. Yet eighteen out of twenty-one
such persons who were interviewed said that they would wish to be
resuscitated in the event of relapse and of their requiring such treatment
to restore their previous state—a result which flies in the face of most
modern mainstream medical and philosophical thought. The authors
quoted Tolstoy: 'The most difficult but the most essential thing is to love
life, to love it even when one suffers—because life is all'. This absolutist
view has been less poetically expressed by saying it may be that death is
the worst of all evils;[5] along with this, it has also been suggested that one
must believe in an after-life if passive involuntary euthanasia is to be
ethically acceptable.[6] Few perhaps would go as far as that; nevertheless,
selective non-treatment must be very much easier for the physician who
holds deep religious convictions which allow him to think in such terms.

Productive and non-productive treatment

Although the foregoing arguments might suggest the reverse, there are
certainly some patients for whom treatment is contraindicated. They
range over the whole therapeutic spectrum, from those who are being
wholly supported by complex machinery—who are discussed in chapter
5—to those whose immediate requirements for treatment would involve
no more than an intramuscular injection of an antibiotic. Decisions as to
what treatment should be given lie in the clinical field; they are technical in nature and it is quite permissible to hold that they should be left
in the hands of those who have the technical expertise—i.e. doctors—
who should be free from outside interference.

Yet, technical decisions of such gravity must be grounded on an
acceptable general ethical base; moreover, the practitioner of selective
non-treatment has not, thus far, been absolved from a seemingly logical
charge of murder. The resolution of both issues may be founded, even if
not entirely satisfactorily, on what has become known as the ordinary/
extraordinary treatment test—a moral test which is generally attributed
to Pope Pius XII. Historically, Roman Catholic theologians have been
the firmest advocates of an absolute sanctity of life ethos. Any modification of that stance which is put forward by the Catholic Church must,
therefore, carry especial weight and will merit careful consideration. The
Pope said:

> Man has a right and duty in the case of severe illness to take the
> necessary steps to preserve life and health. That duty . . . evolves
> from charity as ordained by the Creator, from social justice and
> even from strict law. But he is obliged at all times to employ only
> ordinary means . . . that is to say those means which do not impose
> an extraordinary burden on himself or others.[7]

This obvious departure from a policy of absolute reverence for life appears almost revolutionary. It is, in fact, no more than an authoritative restatement of a doctrine which has been evolving over the centuries starting with Banez in 1595 and one which has received confirmation from the Church as a whole in recent years.[8] The doctrine as propounded by Pope Pius XII is, however, difficult both to explain and to apply because of its generality, and raises the inevitable question: What form of therapy constitutes extraordinary treatment? Does it begin at intensive care, at antibiotic therapy or at intravenous infusion?

To pose such a question is, however, to misunderstand the nature of the test. His Holiness himself qualified 'ordinary' as being 'according to personal circumstances, the law, the times, and the culture'. The test is, therefore, to be looked at not in the context of a choice of possible therapeutic regimes but in the light of the circumstances of the individual patient—it is *he* who is being treated and it is *his* quality of life, not that of the average patient, which dictates the course to be followed.[9] Moreover, it is justifiable to weigh in the balance such variables as the emotional and economic effects on the patient's family. The definition of extraordinary in, say, the United States, may be quite different from that in the United Kingdom and there will be a vast number of variations within each sub-culture which will depend upon the precise conditions surrounding the individual case.

The precept is more easily understood and is perhaps more acceptable if the decision to withhold treatment is couched as a productive/non-productive test—or, more simply, in terms of what will treatment achieve for the patient? It has been argued[10] that to reduce quality of life decisions to what are almost technical problem-solving exercises is to evade substantive moral issues. Many would regard this as being no bad thing insofar as treatment of the individual is inherently pragmatic. Nonetheless, it will be seen that others besides the patient must be involved—for example, the family or those competing for the use of a therapeutic resource—and the better view would surely be that this expanded responsibility calls for decisions to be made within a strong moral framework. It may be human for a family to hope to prevent their inheritance disappearing, for little apparent purpose, into the coffers of an expensive nursing home, but there can be no valid ethical justification for such an attitude. It is in precisely such circumstances that the utilitarian ethos concerning the distribution of happiness breaks down.

The weight of the contribution to decision making which is to be vested in others, such as the physician and the family, is determined by the overriding factor of the patient's condition. We have already discussed the sentient terminally ill patient and, whether or not a competent patient is in the final stages of life, he or she is entitled to refuse or to accept treatment. As Meyers has said,[11] there is no established legal requirement that a competent adult patient with no minor dependents

131,473

must obtain the concurrence of their family members for his therapeutic decision to be valid. Indeed, the law in the United States would seem to be quite the contrary and, in this connection, what holds true in America is also true in the United Kingdom. At the other end of the scale, we have the deeply comatose patient on an artificial life support system, for whom decisions must be made by a surrogate. Somewhere in between, we have the aged patient with a degree of dementia. It is within this last category that the competing interests of the various parties are most difficult to define, and where the moral issues are at their most tender.

The problems of dementia

The inclination of modern philosophers to pre-empt death has already been noted. Once a sizeable body of opinion begins to correlate person-hood or humanity with intellectual function, the elderly become an increasingly endangered group. The moment such phrases as: 'The rest of the body exists in order to support the brain—the brain is the individual'[12] are accepted, people will begin to wonder what may be done about bodies that are supporting a failing brain.

There is no doubt that those who suffer from pre-senile or senile dementia can be very difficult both as relatives and as patients. They tend to be highly suspicious, demanding and, seemingly, ungrateful. To all appearances, their lives are of minimal quality and many outside observers will subscribe to the view that they should end as soon as possible.

But the elderly are still equal persons in law—and the demented are entitled to the same respect from the State as those in full possession of their faculties. The fact that they do not receive it may reflect the fact that they vote only sparingly in proportion to their total numbers and, accordingly, have little political power. It is, therefore, especially important that their needs are well considered by the medical profession. The major barrier to an objective assessment of these needs is that it must be made by those who are young and who are at a disadvantage in understanding the problems of old age. The cussedness of the elderly comes to be regarded as evidence of incapacity; a failure to understand is interpreted as mental incompetence, thereby excluding from con-sideration the possible effect of unsympathetic communication. Rhoads' observation[13]—that the extent to which age is a factor in deciding to relax therapeutic efforts seems to depend somewhat on the age of the physician making the decision—deserves serious consideration.

No one can deny that there is always a case for considering the productivity of treatment in the management of the demented patient but it could be that the case is, currently, being pressed unnecessarily hard. Phrases such as 'death with dignity' may well be empty rhetoric[14] simply because we do not and cannot know how the senile dement sees

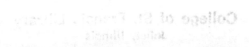

his or her life—the situation is comparable to that of the Down's syndrome baby (see p.61). Every sympathy is due to those who have to look after the elderly but, when it comes to assessing the quality of their lives, care must be taken lest acceptance of the patient's right to die does not lead to an attitude of callousness and helplessness. [15] Veatch has taken the extreme view that 'death is most appropriately thought of as the irreversible loss of the embodied capacity for social interaction'[16] but, even if this is accepted, 'useful' interaction must not be confined to that which would be acceptable to the young and healthy. Pneumonia has been described as the old man's friend; it should never have to be admitted that the truer aphorism is that pheumonia in an old man is his attendants' best friend. [17]

It is worth noting that Campbell, who is a strong supporter of selective treatment has, nevertheless, emphasised that too easy acceptance of the 'person philosophy' could lead to an undesirable therapeutic inertia. [18] Decisions must be reached through what might be called 'due process' and this must be particularly so in the context of surgery for the aged. The surgeon is in a unique relationship insofar as he is unlikely to be in overall charge of the patient. Other than for technical reasons, he cannot withhold surgery purely on the basis of the subject's age and he may well have no knowledge of the patient's total ambience, particularly when he is presented with an emergency situation. On all counts, he has great difficulty in applying the standard ordinary/extraordinary treatment test. [19] The surgeon has fewer options open to him in his choice of treatment and in many ways this simplifies the ethical analysis. Effectively, he is left with a feasibility test: can the operation be done with reasonable safety and probability of success rather than ought it to be done on a quality of life basis? If it is feasible, it should be done except, of course, in the face of a rational refusal. The practice of passive euthanasia would, therefore, seem to be a problem for geriatric medicine rather than for geriatric surgery.

Passive euthanasia and the law

The emphasis throughout this section has, thus far, been on the thought and care which must be applied to selective non-treatment. It may be that mistakes will be made—prognosis is no less difficult to establish than is diagnosis—but they will be made in good faith and with beneficence to the patient as the primary motive. The death of the patient may be intended and effected but there is no 'malice aforethought' or, in Scots terms, 'evil intent'. As a result, I do not believe that withholding therapy can be looked upon as equal to murder. But that does not necessarily establish that causing death in this way is not unlawful; the practice still has to be justified legally.

It is a feature of the law in all common law countries that omissions are treated as being different from commissions. It is possible to commit an

offence by omission only when there is a legal duty to act. How this
affects the doctor is nowhere stated in unequivocal terms but the general
view that a physician is entitled to give up treatment when he thinks it is
of no practical value is widely accepted. His duty is to make reasonable
efforts while maintaining regard for customary practice and expectations. [20]

While some might hold that uncertainty is an unsatisfactory condition, others would contend that the status quo operates well. [21] In
addition it is true that decisions not to treat are taken routinely
world-wide. 'The medical profession' said Ormrod in 1977, [22] '[has]
implicitly accepted the concept of 'quality of life' from which it has, in
the past, always fought shy'. There can, thus, be no question of the
criminal prosecution of a practice which is incontrovertibly accepted
within the profession. On the assumption that the acceptance is one
which is *rightly* made, [23] legal intervention is likely only when treatment
is of a technically advanced nature and the decision over terminating it
raises questions of activity rather than of simple non-prescription. Legal
justification of therapeutic withdrawal becomes more blurred when the
duty of treatment, which is essentially a clinical matter, becomes confused with the duty of care, which is a legal concept. This potential
conflict is well illustrated in the context of feeding.

Feeding as an aspect of treatment

There are extreme views as to the relationship between feeding and
treatment. One is that the former is an integral part of the latter and, as
such, is subject to the same tests of clinical judgment; the other is that
feeding is a basic human duty and that failure to supply nourishment
must be neglect—possibly, criminal neglect.

So far as is known, the matter has been publicly aired in the United
Kingdom only in relation to the neonate. The case of *Arthur* is discussed
in chapter 6. Here it need only be said that, following that case, it is
unlikely that instructions not to feed a newborn will be given in future in
the absence of good *physical* reasons for so doing. Further, the indications
are that the practice of not feeding an infant which is substandard only by
reason of its mental state is currently illegal in the United States, Canada
and Australia. Feeding of the aged and of the terminally ill has, however,
become a burning and, so far, unresolved issue in the United States.

A difficulty which extends throughout the feeding debate is that of
definition. The provision of nourishment runs from simple spoon feeding, through using the nasal tube and intravenous line to gastrostomy,
which involves moderately severe surgery. There are, therefore, good
reasons for weighing up the risks of the procedure should the question of
the propriety of artificial feeding arise. These considerations were particularly well demonstrated in the celebrated Californian case involving
Drs Barber and Nejdl. [24] These physicians, having come to a clinical

decision and having conferred with the relatives, removed respirator support and both nasogastric and intravenous feeding lines from a patient who was in what would have been described in Britain as the persistent vegetative state (see p.44); the doctors were indicted for murder when their patient died.

The subsequent history of the case was particularly turbulent. The charge was dismissed in the Magistrate's Court but was revived on appeal by the prosecution. The doctors, in turn, appealed against the reinstatement of their case and it was only after this hearing that the matter was finally dropped. In the course of the appeal hearing, the court found their behaviour to have been justified in that treatment was, by this time, ineffective. More importantly in the present context, it was determined that artificial feeding was part of that treatment and could be terminated on the same grounds of being ineffective or unproductive. This would seem now to be the agreed principle throughout the United States.

But it is a principle which has been established only after much debate and one which may still be, to an extent, undecided. In the case of Conroy, which arose in the Eastern state of New Jersey, court permission was sought, and granted, to remove a nasogastric tube from a patient who was demented, gravely ill physically and unable to swallow, but who was not comatose. The reasons the court gave for agreeing to the cessation of feeding included their acceptance that the patient had been irrevocably reduced to a very primitive intellectual level and that, therefore, there was no valid purpose to be served by employing active treatment designed to prolong life. Her doctor's contention that it was contrary to his medical ethics to remove the tube was rejected. The decision of the trial court was appealed and, although Ms Conroy had, by then, died from natural causes, the Court of Appeal reversed the decision. [25]

This reversal was based on the assumption that, had the nasogastric tube been withdrawn, the patient would have died from a new condition—dehydration and starvation; she would, therefore, have been actively killed. The New Jersey Court of Appeal clearly considered that, in the particular circumstances of the case, they were being asked to condone active euthanasia and they could find no basis for doing so. They were also concerned lest the principle should be extended and seriously affect the treatment of the mentally retarded and of the senile demented—and this, as has been discussed already and will be reverted to later, is a matter for very real concern. The Supreme Court of New Jersey, however, reversed the decision of the Appeal Court[26] and did so largely on the grounds that feeding was a form of therapy which the patient was entitled to refuse, such refusal being competent, when appropriate, through the medium of a guardian. Even so, the Supreme Court also showed great anxiety that the grounds for such decisions should be strictly contained. The conditions laid down in the absence of any indication of the patient's wishes were that it should be clear that the

burden of continued life with treatment outweighed the benefits of that
life and that the recurring, unavoidable and severe pain of the patient's
life with treatment should be such that the effect of administering
life-sustaining treatment would be inhumane.

In so saying, the court specifically deemed it inappropriate that a
guardian should be empowered to determine that the patient's life was
not worth living simply because the 'quality' of that life or his value to
society seemed negligible to the guardian. 'The mere fact that a patient's
functioning is limited or his prognosis is dim', said Schreiber J, 'does not
mean that he is not enjoying what remains of his life or that it is in his
best interest to die . . . More wide-ranging powers to make decisions
about other people's lives . . . would create an intolerable risk for socially
isolated and defenseless people suffering from physical or mental handicaps'. This opinion, to which there was only one judicial dissent, runs
contrary to most legal thought in the United States but it strongly
reinforces the need for caution, which has already been noted, in making
these assessments.

Several other feeding cases have been reviewed in the American
courts[27] but these are more appropriately considered in the context of
suicide (see chapter 4). But from what has already gone, it can be
suggested that a distinction is being made between invasive and non-
invasive feeding methods. Invasive methods involve therapeutic expertise and can, therefore, be regarded properly as being part of treatment;
the likelihood of useful recovery can be taken into account in the
management of the patient. Invasive procedures would certainly include
gastrostomy and intravenous feeding. The appeal court in *Conroy* considered the nasogastric tube to be no more than a simple device which is
part of routine nursing care and whose use does not constitute medical
treatment. They have not experienced the tribulations of a newly qualified house-officer attempting a technique for the first time. In contrast, I
would classify the tube as being invasive as did the Supreme Court in
Conroy—the difference of opinions however, indicates the difficulties
inherent in drawing this kind of distinction. At the other end of the scale
there is normal spoon feeding which is clearly non-invasive, is part of
basic nursing care and cannot be considered as being subject to therapeutic privilege. Yet, even here, shades of grey appear—how much
force, for example, can be used to feed a recalcitrant patient orally before
the process becomes invasive?[28]

In the end, it seems possible only to lay down the minimum requirement which is that nutrition and hydration should never be withheld
from a patient who is able to take them normally by mouth. No arguments as to the quality of life should be allowed to obscure this basic
principle of humanity. This is implied by Meyers[29] in his summing up:
'The greater the invasiveness and the more hopeless the prognosis, the
less will be the obligation to provide other than misting and manual

feeding by mouth'. Withdrawal of the last facilities are not even considered.

Active involuntary euthanasia

Active involuntary euthanasia involves taking the life of a person who has not indicated any such desire—and, indeed, of one who may positively wish to live. It represents the ultimate denial of the sanctity of life ethos and it is difficult to see how it can subsist within a framework of ethical medical practice. Involuntary euthanasia strikes at the heart of personal autonomy and its justification through the utilitarian ethic is arguable only on very tenuous grounds, if, at all. The only way in which one can attempt to justify a doctor taking the life of a patient deliberately and on his own initiative is by extending a principle which has already been shown to be morally acceptable. Thus, having acknowledged that it may be ethical to allow a patient to die by withdrawing or withholding life-saving treatment in well defined circumstances, it is possible to argue that the same patient's benefit would be better served by painless extermination—indeed, such extrapolation follows inexorably from any premise that killing and letting die are of the same order. Alternatively, it might be possible to, so to speak, turn the doctrine of double effect on its head and contend that the most effective way to kill pain is to kill the person suffering that pain. This involves accepting that it is morally permissible to achieve a good result from a bad act. Although this lies outside the true definition of the doctrine, it can be done while still maintaining purity of intent. But, once either proposition is accepted, it is undeniable that an incremental step has been taken towards an act which is morally untenable—that is, killing a patient from motives other than his own best interests. In other words, we have introduced the wedge—or slippery slope effect.

It is hard to understand how anyone who has watched the escalation of abortion can deny the reality of the wedge effect and the possibility of its application to other contentious areas of medical practice. Nevertheless, the 'slippery slope' theory has always been, and remains, unpopular. Williams,[30] admittedly many years ago, was particularly critical of the wedge argument on the grounds that there is no human conduct from which evil cannot be imagined to follow if it is persisted in when some of the circumstances are changed. The elements of escalation are, however, implicit in the pro-euthanasia stance. Williams quoted several passages from Lord Dawson in the 1950 parliamentary debates:[31]

> I would say that this is a courageous age, but it has a different set of values from the ages which have gone before. It looks upon life more from the point of view of quality than of quantity. It places less value on life when its usefulness has come to and end . . . There has gradually crept into medical opinion . . . the feeling that we should make the act of dying more gentle and peaceful even if it does

involve curtailment of the length of life . . .

and later:

> When the gap between life hindered by incurable disease and death becomes wider . . . there is in the aggregate an unexpressed growth of feeling that the shortening of the gap should not be denied when the real need is there. This is due, not to a diminution in courage, but rather to a truer conception of what life means and what the end of its usefulness deserves.

All of which may be unexceptional but remains faintly disturbing in its potential. In discussing the possibility that a person who has taken life lawfully will then feel less concerned at taking life unlawfully, Williams said that it was ridiculous to imply such an attitude to a physician who gently and humanely extinguishes his patient's life as the last service he can perform for him.

But is it so ridiculous? It may well be asked whether there is any essential difference, other than, perhaps, a degree of knowledge, separating the doctor from any other humane and caring person; and is there no room in the physician's psyche for incremental shifts in motivation? Ironically, it seems that Lord Dawson himself has demonstrated the possibility. We are now informed[32] that he deliberately ended the life of King George V and that this was not done primarily to ease pain but, rather, to ensure a respectable press coverage of his death. Few will have seen the actual relevant document but, on the facts reported, it is difficult to regard this action as anything other than appalling. It is said, no doubt rightly, that the King's life was shortened only by a matter of hours, but it takes little imagination to conceive of further incursions of similar nature and of greater significance occurring in the future. Lord Dawson's action strongly reinforces the views of those who oppose euthanasia legislation for fear of the 'slippery slope'.

Rightly or wrongly, it is on these purely practical grounds that I would reject the suggestion that active and passive euthanasia are indistinguishable. It is also impossible to evade the additional emotional dimension. There can be no doubt that a distinction exists at this level and it is supported, for example, when one reads newspaper reports of the death sentence being carried out in the United States by means of injection.[33] Whether or not their reasoning is logical, very few doctors are prepared to place themselves in the position of 'Dr Death'.[34] It is fair to say that British doctors, as a whole, have not supported euthanasia legislation in the past, the current policy of the British Medical Association being that euthanasia is unacceptable to the profession.[35] The main reaon for this is the effect a legal euthanasia policy might have on the doctor/patient relationship. The likelihood is that this would be profound even if legal termination of life was limited to action requested by the patient and which was consensual in the fullest sense. The position has been summarised admirably by Capron[36] writing as a potential patient:

I never want to have to wonder whether the physician coming into my hospital room is wearing the white coat (or the green scrubs) of a healer—concerned only to relieve my pain and restore me to health—or the black hood of the executioner. Trust between patient and physician is simply too important and too fragile to be subjected to this unnecessary strain.

Yet it seems that medical ethics are seldom static. Thus, we read in 1986[37] that nearly eighty per cent of doctors in one region of the Netherlands have direct experience of euthanasia and that some have deliberately courted prosecution by stating 'active euthanasia' as the cause of death. Equally significant, almost all of those who *have* been prosecuted have been acquitted, indicating public sympathy. As to which, it may be pointed out that jurors are generally not geriatric and that persons in chronic pain will certainly be excused jury service. Those in the prime of life are assessing reactions to a quality of life of which they have no experience.

The ethical shift is, however, not confined to the liberal ambience of the Netherlands. In the same article, it is noted that the British Medical Association is being asked by its members to reconsider its policy. Nowhere is it positively suggested that *involuntary* euthanasia should be legalised but it is the direction—of 'an uncontrolled movement towards including intentional killing in the range of therapeutic options'—which is disturbing.

It is also possible to make a moral distinction between active and passive involuntary euthanasia on the grounds that, in the former, the doctor is arrogating to himself almost superhuman powers of diagnosis and prognosis; active killing allows of no second thoughts. Fundamentally, anyone who engages in active involuntary euthanasia is stripping the subject of his or her last vestige of autonomy and is, thereby, acting immorally.

There remain the legal constraints and, here, the position in the United Kingdom is clear—deliberate killing within the medical framework is illegal, with or without the consent of the patient. Even so, both intent and causation are difficult to demonstrate in the event of a criminal prosecution and it was for this reason that the charge was one of attempted murder in the 1986 case of *R v Carr*—which is, so far as I know, the only truly relevant case to have come before the British courts.

Dr Carr was acquitted—a massive dose of barbiturates was given accidentally—but, during his summing-up, Mars-Jones J had this to say:

> However gravely ill a man may be, however near his death he is, he is entitled in our law to every hour, nay every minute of life that God has granted him. That hour or hours may be the most precious and most important hours of a man's life. There may be business to transact, gifts to be given, forgivenesses to be said, attitudes to be

expressed, farewells to be made, 101 bits of unfinished business which have to be conducted.[38] The ultimate rejection of involuntary euthanasia is founded on its inherent assumption of paternalistic privilege. Mars-Jones' words are as good an expression of this rejection as is likely to be recorded.

Other 'mercy killing'

The doctor may not be the only person who can, with some justification, feel the need to end a suffering patient's life. The sick are not always hospitalised—there may simply be no facilities available or the condition, particularly if of a mental and congenital nature, may not be amenable to treatment. In these circumstances, relatives who are providing care at home may also sense that a life is useless and may be tempted into what is commonly known as 'mercy killing'.

In many ways, it is possible to feel greater sympathy with such persons than with the doctor. They have accepted a duty rather than passing their obligations on to local authorities and thereby condemning their charges to institutions of varying, and often poor, quality; they are commonly isolated and have no ancillary help to relieve a constant burden; they have little knowledge of pharmacology and therapy; and, perhaps most important of all, any lethal action they may feel constrained to take is, in contrast to that taken by the doctor, almost certain to be discovered.

Relatives who kill for 'mercy' are, therefore, almost always to be regarded as being at the end of their tether. They are certainly not insane but it is easy to see their faculties as being so disturbed as to place them in a different category from murderers. There have been intermittent attempts to introduce 'mercy killing' as a legal category of homicide but the opposition has always been strong. To quote from Williams:

> The Criminal Law Revision Committee in its working paper . . . proposed an offence of mercy killing . . . but this met with intense opposition from Christian bodies and societies . . . so the proposal disappeared without trace in the final Report.[39]

Despite this, most people would not wish to see genuine 'mercy killers' sentenced to imprisonment for life. Strictly speaking, it is difficult to plead diminished responsibility in such cases, in that it has been held that, to satisfy the Homicide Act 1957, s.2(1), there must be a state of mind which is so different from that of ordinary human beings that the reasonable man would term it abnormal.[40] Rather, it is often the case that the killing, when it occurs, has been responsibly considered and is fully intended.[41] Moreover, it is a regrettable fact that unethical motives for the early demise of relatives do exist. For all these reasons, 'mercy killings' are generally brought to trial. In obvious cases, the prosecution may pre-empt the jury by charging manslaughter, or culpable homicide, only; otherwise, they may either accept such a plea as an alternative to murder or the possibility that such a verdict will be left to the jury who may well be predisposed to a liberal interpretation of the Homicide Act 1957—an interpretation which is often assisted by equally sympathetic attitudes on the part of psychiatrists who may stretch the limits of the diagnosis of depressive psychosis. In all such cases, the court may then reflect its appreciation of the individual case in sentencing[42]—none of which diminishes the importance that the law attaches to the preservation of life. What it does is to offer a quality of legal response to an understandable, albeit still illegal, assessment of the quality of life.

4. Suicide

The pathological condition of depressive psychosis is the dominant regulator of suicide rates; self-killing within this condition is no more than the last phase of the disease and cannot be regarded as voluntary. Suicide by choice, however, has a history which has varied both with time and with geography. Some traditional bases for suicide were no more than a choice between that form of death and execution—as in the well-known Grecian tradition. In other instances, suicide can be said to involve an evaluation of the emotional quality of life to which death may seem preferable. 'Taking the honourable way out' in a Western setting may be more a fantasy of Victorian novels than a cultural reality but there can be no doubt that it was, and probably still is, a genuine code of behaviour in, for example, sections of Japanese society.

Taking one's own life voluntarily is, however, a direct challenge to the sanctity of human life ethos and something which has been consistently condemned by Christian and other monotheistic religions. Such action is supposedly an unforgivable interference with the will of God. Quite why suicide was viewed in this way rather than being looked upon as a legitimate use of God-given free-will is difficult to understand. Nevertheless, because the law of the person was so firmly based on ecclesiastical precepts, suicide, together with attempted suicide, was considered to be not only a religious but also a secular crime until 1961. The continued association of criminality with what was, by the twentieth century, essentially a private matter was, however, incompatible with growing public awareness of and sensitivity to personal autonomy; suicide was removed from the list of criminal offences by the Suicide Act 1961 (appendix C). Aiding and abetting suicide remains a serious offence under s.2 of the Act and that, as is discussed later, is of considerable significance for the doctor. It is worth pointing out that the Suicide Act 1961 does not cover Scotland where it is probable that suicide was not regarded as being criminal at the time the Act was passed;[1] the logical corollary is that there is no such offence as abetment of suicide in Scotland and the later discussion must be read with that qualification in mind.

The Suicide Act 1961 was the first English statute, other than the strictly limited Infant Life (Preservation) Act 1929, to admit of exceptions to a sanctity of life rule. It has wide application but here we are concerned, in the main, with those aspects of suicide which involve the practice of medicine.

Many of these have already been addressed in or can be implied from the discussion of terminal illness and euthanasia. There can be no doubt as to the competent patient's right to refuse treatment for a lethal condition but there is considerable doubt, both in the United Kingdom and in the United States, as to whether this constitutes suicide in legal terms. Any distinction is now more a point of academic debate than of practical importance—the intention is to die.[2] A person is also entitled to refuse remedial treatment of a primary suicidal attempt. No matter how much he might wish to do so, a doctor who sutures an incised radial artery, or who initiates gastric lavage, commits an assault if he acts against the expressed wishes of the patient. Clearly, however, he is in a moral dilemma of outstanding proportions. He may accept that he has a legal justification to 'pass by on the other side'. Alternatively, in an effort to salve his own conscience—and the greater part of ethical medical practice is founded upon conscience—he may well plead necessity; he may reasonably assume that the patient is, in fact, not competent and so adopt the cover of therapeutic privilege. He may wait until the patient is comatose and then suppose that there has been a change of mind on his or her part. In any event, successful treatment may receive little thanks and may, indeed, attract opprobrium—for it has been said that 'the Good Samaritan is a character unesteemed by the English law'.[3] Despite this, it is thought that the legal response to non-consensual interference in suicide would be likely to be favourable to the doctor in the United Kingdom[4] and the courts might be even more sympathetic in the United States where the State not only has a compelling interest in the prevention of suicide but where a clinical assessment of mental incompetence would carry great weight.[5] The doctor's quandary in this context is, perhaps, at its most acute when related to suicide by starvation.[6] This may arise in a political or quasi-political setting or may be one facet of a general refusal to take medical advice and treatment.

The suicidal political hunger strike places the doctor in an almost intolerable situation insofar as the office of prison medical officer carries with it both a professional duty to the prisoners and an administrative allegiance to the authorities. Current British governmental instructions as to the forced feeding of hunger-strikers are that the medical officer should first satisfy himself that the prisoner's capacity for rational judgment is unimpaired by mental or physical illness; the prisoner must be told that he will continue to receive medical supervision and advice, that food will be made available, and that he will be removed to the prison hospital if necessary. At the same time, he must be clearly warned that the consequent deterioration in his health may be allowed to continue without medical intervention unless he specifically requests it.[7]

All of which seems clear and in accord with the Declaration of Tokyo 1975 which is concerned with 'torture and other cruel, inhuman or

degrading treatment or punishment in relation to detention and imprisonment'. That is, until it is added that individual medical officers still
have the right to force feed if they consider that it will be beneficial—an
outcome which is certainly to be expected, particularly if the person is
too weak to resist. Politicians are thus unwilling to lay down a political
rule which would interfere in a doctor/patient relationship—albeit one
of an unusual character. Effectively, the doctor is expected to make a life
or death decision but to do this in the knowledge that, whichever way his
decision goes, it is bound to have repercussions—possibly including
further loss of life—which are beyond his control and, indeed, beyond
his competence to assess. Zellick has also pointed out how unjustly
diverse the results of such an equivocal directive may be. Fortunately,
these problems have to be resolved very rarely. One senses, again, a
different approach being adopted in the United States where the concept
of the State's obligation to protect the health and welfare of persons in its
care and custody is still deeply held.[8] The courts have approved force
feeding of prisoners who have, *inter alia*, used self-starvation as a method
by which to draw attention to conditions in under-developed countries[9]
or because death was thought to be preferable to a life in prison.[10] It is
doubtful, however, whether such orders would be made in the face of
recognised political or religious conviction.[11]

Self-starvation as part of refusal of medical assistance does not seem to
have been addressed in Britain but there have been a number of interesting court decisions in the United States. Patients have themselves, or
through guardians, authorised essential feeding lines to be removed, the
general theme being that non-productive feeding is as rejectable as is
non-productive therapy. In what is, perhaps, the most extreme case
reported, the court conceded that a disabled yet viable patient was not
only entitled to end her poor quality of life by self-starvation but could
expect assistance from the medical staff in so doing.[12]

This unusual case leads us back to the more mundane consideration of
the doctor's role when his patient, suffering from terminal or painful
illness, wishes to end an apparently intolerable life—the classic voluntary euthanasia situation which is, in practice, indistinguishable from
suicide.

Voluntary active euthanasia

There is no problem as to whether a patient may take an overdose of
drugs or remove his arteriovenous shunt without fear of the law—it is
plain that he may, so long as his action has no direct effect on others.
Whether he may do so morally is less certain. I have already indicated my
belief that, given the right circumstances and motivation, it may be
perfectly possible to equate an acceptance of suicide with a belief in a
creator-God—the 'sinfulness' of suicide seems to be something of a
human artefact. But since the matter depends so much on individual

conscience, generalisation is useless.

The question of whether the doctor or nursing staff has an obligation to prevent suicide has been partially discussed (p.28). The hospital environment is, however, unique and whatever the legal niceties it would be an unusual and, perhaps, foolhardy staff which stood by and watched a successful suicide attempt. Apart from any ethical considerations, the publicity attached to a Coroner's inquest or to an inquiry held under the Fatal Accident and Sudden Deaths Inquiry (Scotland) Act 1976 would be unlikely to be favourable; moreover, there would be a strong possibility of an action for negligence being brought either by relatives or by the patient himself in the event of failure. Such an action would, however, be on the basis of negligent treatment, through inadequate supervision, of a patient suffering from depressive psychosis.[13] That is an entirely different situation from one in which the patient is making a rational decision; intervention would always be expected in the presence of mental disorder. Even in the event of an autonomous choice being exercised, it is difficult to see how the doctor could not be both legally and morally bound to attempt to dissuade the patient from his projected course and, further, to remove, so far as possible, any opportunity for carrying it out. Conditions might, however, be difficult and it was in the hope of resolving doubts that the unsuccessful Incurable Patients Bill 1976 proposed that: 'No person shall be under any duty to interfere with any course of action taken by an incurable patient to relieve his suffering in a manner likely to cause his own death and any interference intentionally undertaken contrary to the known wishes of the patient shall be unlawful'. As has been discussed already, it may well be that such legislation is unnecessary—and it could be unacceptable to the doctor who is committed to the sanctity of life in all circumstances.

Suicide and attempted suicide having been removed from the list of criminal offences, it is inevitable that those contemplating the deed may now feel free to seek assistance. There could be occasions when the doctor who, believing in the quality of life doctrine, might feel that it was right and proper for him to help and, carried to its logical conclusion, this line of reasoning would allow the doctor to inject the lethal contents of a syringe into the vein of a patient who had asked him to do so. The law here is perfectly clear and rests on two principles. The first of these is intent. Motive is of no consequence if the intention to kill is there and the victim is killed. Secondly, consent cannot decriminalise a serious crime and, except in the very circumscribed case of double suicide pacts, intentional killing carries the risk of a charge of manslaughter at least.[14] This possibility is however, excessively rare in practice. It is far more likely that the doctor will be asked to provide the means of suicide without actually administering it and, at this point, the correct interpretation of the law seems rather less obvious.

Assisted suicide

The scenario commonly envisaged is that the doctor, having been asked by the patient, gives him information as to the lethal dose of a drug and leaves such a dose within his reach. The question then arises as to whether the doctor, in agreeing to do so, commits an offence against the Suicide Act 1961, s.2 which involves aiding, abetting, counselling, or procuring a suicide—an offence which, incidentally, carries a sentence of up to fourteen years' imprisonment.

It is probable that such a procedure would not constitute abetment because the offence requires presence at the scene and some element of active participation. Judicial practice however, is, to consider aiding, abetting, counselling and procuring as a whole and it is difficult to see how the process could fail to constitute counselling and procuring: 'a person procures a thing by setting out to see that it happens and taking the appropriate steps to produce that happening',[15] and that is precisely what has been done. Nevertheless, Professor Furmston[16] has used the interesting illustration of a patient dependent upon a respirator. It would, he said,

> be hazardous [for the doctor] to switch off a support system simply because an alert intelligent person, though in great pain, wishes to be 'switched off'. Obviously, if you put him near enough to the switch so that he can switch it off himself, that would seem to be alright.[17]

This would suggest that the significant criminal element might be counselling—everyone knows how to operate an electric switch without coaching. By analogy, there would then be no offence in leaving a lethal dose with a person who understood drug dosage and actions but the reverse might hold if the facts had to be explained. To introduce such pedantry however, is only to demonstrate the degree of sophistry and evasion which pervades this area of debate. Kennedy,[18] for example, has observed that the court would probably believe the doctor if he contended that the pills had been intended for ensuring sleep and this pragmatic view may well be correct—in practice, no doctor has been prosecuted under s.2. Even so, it is less than satisfactory that the law should depend upon such blatant circumvention.

An attempt to anticipate the doctor's position by reference to that of non-medics is, similarly, unrewarding. Prosecutions for abetting suicide are occasionally brought but are rarely reported and the impression is that, in the circumstances envisaged, sentencing would be very light— Williams has, indeed, pointed to the near absurdity of attributing criminality to abetment of a non-criminal act.[19] This would not necessarily be so were the would-be suicide a young, fit person: the intent, as well as the motive, might then be suspect. Similarly, the law might take a different view of attempts to disseminate a way of thought, or provide 'counsel', to a wider public. The precedents in this last respect are, again, helpful only in a negative sense. All that can be said is that abetment continues to be a very narrowly defined concept. Effectively, there can be no aiding or abetting unless the action is directed at a specific person who is known to be contemplating taking his or her own life;[20] but this does not tell us when distance becomes proximity.

It would be nice to be able to say that, irrespective of the law, the propriety of what is commonly called 'leaving the pills' could be determined on ethical principles but even here there is no unanimity. Directly opposing views can be defended equally well. On the one hand, it can be held that the doctor who administers a lethal dose on request allows no time for reflection and is, to that extent, usurping the patient's freedom of choice. Merely providing the means, however, preserves the patient's autonomy and ensures a true, fully considered 'consent' to suicide, and there is much to be said for this approach. The alternative is to see the doctor who assists passively in voluntary euthanasia but who declines to do so actively as being guilty of moral cowardice. He is, so to speak, accepting the fact but is washing his hands of responsibility and, as I have suggested elsewhere,[21] Pontius Pilate remains a doubtful moral authority.

It can only be concluded that assisting in suicide is so much a matter of individual professional conscience—which may, in turn, be influenced by the minutiae of the circumstances—that it is impossible to reach an acceptable consensus. It may well be asked also whether, in practice, the problem is not one which is emptier of significance than appears. Many eminent professionals will, when speaking unofficially, pay lip-service to the fact that assisted suicide occurs in a medical setting. Nevertheless, I cannot remember ever seeing it, or hearing directly of it, being practised; indeed, the conditions in a hospital setting are such that the chances of a conscientious objector, or even a normally efficient associate, interfering with the plan are great enough to make one doubt if it could succeed. 'Leaving the pills' would seem to be a problem, if there is one, of private domiciliary or nursing home practice—and, even then, one of the 1950s rather than the 1980s.

5. Brain Damage and Death

Thus far, the discussion has concentrated mainly on terminal or intolerable illness suffered by competent and sentient patients. The definitive points have been not only that the patients were able to express themselves but also that they could do so in the light of past experience and of considered expectations for the future.

Similarly, the doctors involved have had a standard by which to assess the patient's current quality of life and have, in general, been able to say that, bad as that standard now is, it can only deteriorate in the future. This section will extend the debate into the more difficult ambit of the incompetent patient and, particularly, of those incompetents who are suffering from an illness which is acute and incapacitating but within which some sort of life can be maintained by modern technology—we are, in fact, entering the ill-defined area of non-voluntary euthanasia. There are several variant models which could be used but, for the sake both of clarity and brevity, I propose to illustrate the theme only through the medium of the seriously brain-damaged child or adult.

Incapacitating brain damage can have natural or unnatural causes. The common link between all forms of coma is cerebral hypoxia—shortage of oxygen to the brain—and this, in turn, may derive from many conditions which include: failure of the heart to oxygenate the brain; lesions which occupy space in the unyielding skull and thus cause compression of the blood vessels; direct injury; toxic effects, most commonly associated with the narcotic drugs which act by inhibiting the uptake of oxygen by the nerve cells; and a lack of oxygen in the respiratory atmosphere. Thus, it will be seen that brain damage can occur at any age. Cerebral tumours and prolonged cardiac resuscitation are examples of causes in later adult life while spontaneous subarachnoid haemorrhage or direct injury can cover the whole life span from birth to senescence. Note also that most of the causative conditions are of unnatural type—including, in particular, the inadequate provision of oxygen during poorly administered anasthesia. Such conditions are likely to attract medico-legal attention in their own right.

The brain, the persona and the diagnosis of death

Some simple clinical concepts must be recapitulated because it is impossible to develop either legal or moral theories in this area without some basic understanding of the pathophysiology involved.

The life of the tissues depends on oxygen which is harvested from the air by the lungs and distributed to the tissues by the heart. The heart and lungs are, therefore, mutually dependent—the heart muscle cannot function without oxygen and the distribution of oxygen cannot proceed in the absence of an efficient pulmonary blood circulation. For these reasons, it has been customary to define death in terms of irreversible failure of the cardio-respiratory system or, consequently, as a permanent state of tissue anoxia. This concept can, however, be invalidated by modern techniques. It is often not difficult to restart a heart which has apparently ceased to beat and the function of the lungs can be replaced by machines—either by a respirator which replicates the chest muscle movement or by a ventilator which forces air into the lungs when it cannot be drawn in naturally. The apparently simple conventional distinction between life and death is, thus, put into question.

While the heart is, to an extent, an autonomous organ, the lungs depend on the respiratory centre in the brain stem for their subconscious action; the brain itself is that organ of the body which is most sensitive to oxygen lack and the brain, as a whole, is irreplaceable by machine.[1] Physiologically, therefore, it is possible, and attractive, to define death in terms of brain function rather than of cardio-respiratory integrity. The concept also finds philosophical favour:

> The rest of the body exists in order to support the brain. The brain is the individual . . .[2]

or, as Lord Scarman has put it,

> There is much to be said for the view that life, so far as our species is concerned, is the life of man in a sapient state.[3]

But although Lord Scarman himself was immediately aware of the possibility, this attitude introduces grave moral and legal considerations. The effects of hypoxia on the brain cells are irreparable but the continuing process of destruction is halted when oxygen is resupplied. Along with this, the brain can, for practical purposes, be divided into three areas—the cortex which controls human life, the thalamus which is roughly responsible for our animal existence and the brain stem which controls the various vegetative functions, including that of respiration. These areas are not equally sensitive to oxygen deprivation—the brain stem can withstand a hypoxic insult better than can the thalamus while the cortex is the least resistant. It follows that a person whose brain has been damaged and who has been re-oxygenated will suffer from a degree of residual injury which may run from minor intellectual impairment to obliteration of the brain stem and, with it, the essential respiratory centre—at which point, life of any sort becomes impossible save through the medium of artificial respiration.

The various degrees of hypoxic brain damage—ranging from *coma vigile*, or diminished consciousness to *coma depassé*, or something beyond coma—were first described by French neurologists.[4] The term 'brain death', which was the equivalent of the French *coma dépassé*, was originally coined in the USA in 1971[5] but, in the meantime, the Harvard school had defined what they called 'irreversible coma'.[6] This term introduced an unfortunate semantic confusion because, while the Beecher Committee (1968) were clearly defining what was later to be known as 'brain death', the term 'irreversible coma' implies something less than death and also has a strong conceptual affinity with what the Glasgow workers Jennett and Plum called the 'persistent vegetative state'.[7] In this state, which may last for months or even years, the patient's cerebral cortex is destroyed—he is able to breathe and his heart beats but he will be otherwise insentient.

Thus the quality of existence is altered when some parts of the brain are dead and this, in turn, depends upon the intensity of the hypoxic insult. It cannot, however, be over-stressed that an absolute distinction must be drawn between life, whatever its quality, and death. There are many practical reasons why the concept of brain death or brain stem death should be acceptable to the public. Anything which distracts from that acceptability must be eliminated so far as is possible. In particular, there is no place for such relative assessments as being 'at death's door' or, more emphatically, being 'as good as dead'.[8]

There are two specific areas of concern to be decided in this connection. The first is to distinguish clearly between the persistent vegetative state described by Jennett, and brain death. Unfortunately, there has been some confusion on this point in legal minds—at least in the past. Suggestions have been made that vegetative cases could be used as organ donors[9] and other eminent writers appear to have confused the two conditions.[10] Lord Edmund-Davies has said that:

> Many doctors now regard as dead a patient who is in a state of deep and irremediable unconsciousness even though his heart still beats and he still draws breath.[11]

With all respect, I do not believe this is so; and, if some doctors do hold this view, then they could justly be regarded as being wrong. The persistent vegetative state is one of the most distressing conditions known to medicine, but the profession will be treading shaky ground if it comes to believe that a patient who breathes spontaneously, and supports a heart without mechanical assistance, is not alive. 'But', it will be said, 'a body which has no sentience, no power of choice and no means of communication is no longer a person and has none of the rights of personhood'.[12] I submit that, while this may be impeccable philosophy, it cannot be good medicine. If the proposal is followed through to its logical conclusion, the implications are horrifying. It will be argued later, and also in the following chapter, that there may be good grounds for allowing brain-damaged persons to die; but the basis for this is the interests of the patient, not that he has forfeited his right to life.

The second major dilemma related to the management of the brain damaged raises complex clinical, moral and legal issues. Possibly no-where else in medicine is the question—'given that one can maintain life regardless of its quality, ought one to do so?'[13]—presented so acutely. Variations on the theme are endless but, to ease discussion, I propose to illustrate the difficulties only by reference to the worst possible condi-tions of living—that is, when the brain is so damaged that admission to intensive care is necessary.

Clinical considerations

Before turning to the question of ventilator support, it might be useful to the non-medical reader to distinguish between the respirator and the ventilator; in so doing, the importance of the brain as a measure of the value of human life is emphasised.

The respirator—which used to be known as the 'iron lung'—simulates natural breathing by rhythmic compression and decompression of the chest wall; it is designed for symptomatic treatment of respiratory paralysis resulting from disease of the spinal cord or of peripheral nerves and, accordingly, its use is now almost non-existent in countries where acute anterior poliomyelitis, or 'infantile paralysis', has been virtually eliminated. The practical situation of the patient in a respirator is well-nigh intolerable; he is immobile and is tied to his machine and, yet, as likely as not, he is not only fully conscious but his intellectual capacity is also unaffected. Every instinct tells us that here is a human being in distress who needs our help; moreover, he can live, to a limited extent, in hope. There can have been no doubts within the medical team as to the propriety of instituting respirator treatment, to have failed to do so would have been to watch a conscious person asphyxiate. No one would regard the only available treatment as being extraordinary, still less could therapy which maintains a fully sentient human being be called non-productive. For this reason, were, say, pneumonia to set in, it would be treated without hesitation in the absence of a firm refusal on the part of the patient—and, in point of fact, the vast majority would wish to cling to what others might regard as an unrewarding existence. No one would consider making such an autocratic decision as to turn off the machine and, were such action requested, the chances are it would still not be carried out. This might seem illogical but the situation in which a health carer was asked to asphyxiate his patient inevitably and within a few minutes, would be unique and, in the event of an irreconcilable conflict of opinion, one which would raise a question which would properly be taken to the courts. Yet, insofar as the respirator patient cannot breathe by his own volition, he is less 'alive' by the traditional standards of assessing death than is the brain-damaged patient in the persistent vegetative state. If we apply the same line of thinking to the latter patient, we can see that there would be no hesitation in declining to treat intercurrent pneumonia. Why should there be these differences when neither patient has any prospect of returning to a full life? It must be because we instinctively feel that, ultimately, the quality of life is to be evaluated by reference to the function of the brain.

That distinction having been made, we can turn to the brain-damaged patient on ventilator support. In that state, respiration is replicated by direct cyclical inflation of the lungs—thus, the long term use of the ventilator is limited in practice to the treatment of the unconscious patient.

It is important to distinguish two rather different uses of the ventilator. Every comatose patient who is in incipient respiratory failure may be supported by the ventilator to provide time for diagnosis and assessment. Use of the apparatus can be likened to carrying out laboratory and radiological tests as a prelude to definitive treatment. Following this initial course of action, there are three basic options. The patient can be removed from the ventilator in the knowledge that he will live in an unchanged condition without support; or intensive care can be discontinued in the likelihood that the patient will die—either the condition is seen as being untreatable or prolonged ventilation is regarded as being unproductive care and the patient is left to die in peace; or it can be agreed that the patient's condition is not static, that it may improve and that he should be offered full intensive care. It is this secondary phase which should be regarded as 'admission to the ventilator'.

The decision to admit must be taken in the knowledge that, sooner or later, ventilation has to be discontinued. The critical decision then rests on an assessment of the patient's ultimate condition. For example, is the highest achievement of ventilation likely to be the production of the persistent vegetative state? Although this involves a major exercise in clinical prognosis, the decision also embodies an ethical component. There is much to be said for the view that the ethical aspects of intensive care arise at the *beginning* of treatment and that the dilemmas which appear later in the clinical management of the case all stem from the pivotal act of admission. [14] The situation can be compared, say, to the treatment of strokes in the elderly of whom it has been said:

> Inadequate initial assessment is probably the greatest single cause of inappropriate treatment . . . and may mean a missed opportunity to let dying occur. [15]

Even so, this comment emphasises that the ethical choice, based on the test of treatment productivity depends on clinical expertise: good ethics and good practice are indivisible.

Once it is clear that the patient's condition is not going to improve, there are not only clinical and social indications for withdrawal of treatment but also logistic reasons insofar as scarce resources must be used with maximum efficiency. No resources—whether of apparatus, manpower or finances—are infinite. To retain a non-responsive patient on intensive care is, inevitably, to deprive a potential benefactor of the facility. This unpalatable fact has been expressed:

It is becoming obvious that the costs of the policy [of pursuing the preservation of life] are becoming insupportable.[16]

The Archbishop of Canterbury had the courage to point this out in his Edwin Stevens Lecture in 1977[17]—and received a bad press for so doing. In accepting this principle, and, in practice, it *has* to be accepted, the medical profession must acknowledge the presence of a further weighting factor when assessing the quality of a patient's existence—that is, the quality of the life of others. The problem of how the relative priorities of those competing for treatment are to be judged is extraordinarily difficult to solve. It is not easy to transfer the military concept of triage—or allocating treatment facilities on the basis of the qualitative end result in each case—to civilian life because the vagaries of the latter seldom offer such a well defined aim as winning the battle. I have concluded elsewhere[18] that the only just way of admitting patients to high technology therapy is on the unsatisfactory basis of 'first come, first served'. We are here concerned, however, with withdrawal rather than admission, and two limiting principles can be identified within that concern.

Firstly, once admitted to treatment, a patient cannot be deprived of that treatment simply because another— perhaps more clinically deserving—patient arrives. Secondly, arguments in favour of a decision to re-admit following clinically-based withdrawal must be particularly searching. As to such withdrawal, there are two distinct circumstances in which a clinical decision to stop intensive care of a comatose patient can be properly made—either the treatment has been shown to be no longer productive or the subject is 'brain dead'.

Withdrawal of support from the comatose patient who, although not dead, is not benefiting, involves an agonising decision for the attending physician. But once the die has been cast, there are two possible results: either the patient breathes spontaneously and survives, or he dies as a result of cardio-respiratory failure. The first alternative is illustrated by the well known case of Karen Quinlan[19] and the latter by the Scottish case *Finlayson v HM Adv*[20], both of which will be discussed later. For the present, it need only be said that the decision is essentially a clinical one and one which the doctor is competent to make on the basis of a productive/non-productive treatment test (see p.24). No substantive moral problem arises. There can be no lower quality of life, no greater indignity, no greater suffering for the patient's family than being maintained on intensive care for no other reason than that, although one cannot breathe and will never achieve an improved status, one retains a few reflexes.

Brain dead or brain stem dead?

These considerations apply in even greater force if the patient is, in fact, dead despite the fact that the heart still beats because of pulmonary ventilation. The machine is then ventilating a corpse and, outwith the field of transplantation therapy, there can be very few occasions when it is ethically proper to allow it to do so. Given this premise, the neurosurgeon can terminate treatment without fear of recrimination, and this is the primary value of the concept of brain death. The major remaining point of controversy, however, lies in obtaining organs for transplantation through the medium of the beating heart donor, the question being whether or not the organ donor can truly be said to be dead.

Official recognition of brain death came in two stages in the United Kingdom. In the first,[21] the conference of the Medical Royal Colleges and their Faculties—certainly the greatest concentration of medical expertise available—laid down the diagnostic criteria which consisted, primarily, of the often forgotten conditions for *considering* the diagnosis of brain death and, then, of specific tests for establishing its occurrence. In the second phase,[22] it was agreed that the identification of brain death means that the patient is dead, whether or not the functions of some organs, such as a heartbeat, are still maintained by artificial means.

The semantic and conceptual difficulties arise from the fact that while the conference speaks of brain death, the tests are designed to demonstrate brain stem death. As laid down, they do not test for 'death of the whole brain'; a battery of tests including cerebral angiography and/or the electroencephalogram might go some way to defining the latter but they are not required under the British code of practice.[23] The anomaly is apparent rather than real. The brain stem is that part of the brain which is most resistant to anoxia; it is, therefore, almost inconceivable that the brain stem can be destroyed in the presence of a functioning cerebrum. Very occasionally, a primary lesion arises in the brain stem but this should be clinically diagnosable; otherwise, we are left only with such inappropriate examples as beheading or judicial hanging in which consciousness might persist in the absence of a brain stem.

The majority of British doctors are content with the concept of brain stem death but protests are still raised[24] and will almost certainly continue. Some surgeons will not remove donor organs with the heart still beating and, by disconnecting the life support machine in the operating theatre, they effectively allow the patient to 'die on the table', death then being judged by a flat electrocardiogram. I find this practice illogical in that, if the patient is not considered dead, it is just as improper to 'kill' him as it is to remove his organs. There can be no compromise with the diagnosis of death—a person is either dead or alive and most people are satisfied that, given that the *whole* protocol of testing has been carried out, a person whose brain stem is dead is clinically dead.

Nevertheless, there have been calls for legislation on the matter in the United Kingdom[25] and many of the States in America and Australia, among others, have enacted statutes. The great majority of these define death as being demonstrated either by the irreversible cessation of cardiac and pulmonary function or by the irreversible loss of function of the whole brain.[26] Such statutes are useful in that they clear the air in an area ripe for litigation. By and large, they seem unnecessary but at least they do not make the error of laying down the criteria to be adopted. No past legislation has dictated that a doctor *must* use a stethoscope to diagnose death—he will do so because it is good medical practice. The same reasoning applies in the more unusual condition of diagnosing death through cerebral function. It has been said that: 'the approach that death is essentially a question of clinical judgment is unacceptable'[27] but, like it or not, the diagnosis *is* a clinical exercise to be undertaken in a way which is recognised as valid by reputable medical practitioners.

There remains the moral problem of whether a person who is brain stem dead should continue to be ventilated for reasons other than the transplantation of his or her organs. This problem has manifested itself most commonly in the form of preserving a cadaver's circulation in order to obtain a viable fetus. On the face of things, there is no logical objection to such practice; indeed, the anti-abortionist might hold, with some justification, that there is a positive duty to preserve life when the opportunity arises. Nevertheless, it is equally possible to see the practice as being a dangerous incremental interference with the distinction between life and death—it is not a long step to maintaining ventilation for other much less worthy objectives, such as for life insurance purposes. A more practical objection is that these cases tend to cast further doubts on the validity of the concept of brain stem death. Occasional instances are reported in which the mother has been ventilated for several weeks, a circumstance which is incompatible with Jennett's contention that cardiac function cannot be maintained for more than a few days after death of the brain stem.[28] The possibility is thus raised that the original diagnosis of death was incorrect and this may be associated, at least in part, with a confusion of objectives.

The legal position

The legal response to the removal of life support has been very well illustrated in the United States where many cases are taken to the courts for the solution of what are, essentially, therapeutic decisions. This course of action is rare in the United Kingdom and, as a result, what case law there is tends to come from the criminal courts.

The position in the United Kingdom now seems clear but this conclusion has not been reached without the medical profession facing some difficulties. It is worth considering some of the possible pitfalls. The scene is well set in the words of Kennedy:[29]

> It would be a brave judge who would contemplate with equanimity the headlines of the next day's press proclaiming 'Judge orders burial of man with beating heart'.

While this would be unlikely, it highlights the fact that the doctor, in making the diagnosis of brain stem death, is, effectively, doing much the same thing. There has always been a possibility that some physician might be accused of manslaughter or, even more remotely, of murder.

The distinction between the two turns mainly on whether 'switching off' a life support machine constitutes a commission—that is, a positive act—or merely an omission to treat. Kennedy[30] was of the opinion that it must be classed as an act and likened it to cutting the wire of a tight-rope walker. This view seems acceptable if only on the analogy that you have got to *do* something to turn off the television set. Most writers, however, have been at pains to prove the interpretation of omission and, in the process, have used some interesting illustrations. Williams, for example, compared a machine worked by manual effort with one powered by electricity. Ceasing to crank the former would be an omission, from which he argued that turning off the electricity must be of the same order.[31] Confusion is considerable but the pragmatic, albeit illogical, conclusion is that the inclination of the courts would be to regard the termination of treatment as an omission.

That being so, the question of whether a doctor could be guilty of manslaughter depends on his legal duty to act. It seems self-evident that a doctor who voluntarily undertakes the care of a patient owes that patient a duty and it is worth remembering what Williams has said elsewhere:

> One who deliberately omits to save a life that he is under a legal duty to save is guilty of murder unless the law provides some defence.[32]

The defence of necessity might well be available in this case. Kennedy[33] considered that the doctor discontinuing life support does nothing to warrant a criminal sanction provided he acts in good faith; he bolstered this view by pointing out that anyone else removing support in the conditions envisaged would certainly be guilty of homicide. Against this, Brahams and Brahams[34] believed that allowing a patient to die is a positive malfeasance and, although they were writing in terms of neonates, it is not difficult to extrapolate their views to the adult intensive care unit. Thus, with the legal theorists at some odds, it is as well that there is now some modern case law which has resolved the differences. The prototype case of 1978 is *Finlayson*.[35]

Finlayson was a drug addict who injected his companion with a mixture of narcotic drugs, as a result of which the recipient sustained severe hypoxic brain damage. The victim died shortly after being removed from intensive care on the grounds that improvement in his condition was impossible. Finlayson was charged with culpable homicide and his defence was, in essence, that of *novus actus interveniens*—the doctors, in discontinuing treatment, had broken the logical chain of events and were, in fact, responsible for the proximate cause of death. Note that the victim was described in the opinion of the Appeal Court as being in a 'totally vegetative state'. Whether or not he was 'brain stem dead' in the now accepted sense, the case was decided before the authoritative statement was made that brain stem death represents death of the whole person.[36] In dismissing the appeal against conviction, Lord Justice-General Emslie said:

> Once the initial reckless act causing injury had been committed, the natural consequence which the perpetrator must accept is that the victim's future depended on a number of circumstances, including whether any particular treatment was available, whether it was medically reasonable and justifiable to attempt it and to continue it . . . It certainly cannot be said that the act of disconnecting the machine was an unwarrantable act.

The Scottish case was followed by a similar appeal in England.[37] In two cases following conviction for murder, which were heard simultaneously, the defence was also that the chain of causation had been broken by the discontinuance of intensive care. The medical personnel involved had, by now, the benefit of the Royal Colleges' statement on the diagnosis of death; there can be no doubt that the victims were dead when removed from the ventilator. Lord Lane LCJ was quite positive:

> When a medical practitioner, using generally acceptable methods, came to the conclusion that the patient was for all practical purposes dead, and that all such vital functions as remained were being maintained solely by mechanical means, and accordingly discontinued treatment, that did not break the chain of causation between the initial injury and the death.

The thrust of both judgments is clear. Both opinions (and *Finlayson* was not cited in the English court) relied firmly on the concept of good medical practice. Consequently, it is now reasonable to infer that no doctor would be held criminally liable were he to remove life support on the grounds that it was incapable of improving the patient's quality of life—a quality which was, at the time, abysmal and which could not, on practical grounds, be sustained indefinitely.

That last reservation supports the moral acceptability of the general proposition. Sooner or later, the ventilated patient is bound to contract intercurrent disease, at which point the unproductive treatment test should surely be applied. The purpose in discontinuing useless treatment is to spare the patient unnecessary distress; academic argument as to the positive or negative nature of the action is sterile. A Roman Catholic commentary on this condition is interesting:

> We are to be valued for our personhood and if treatment cannot offer substantial benefit to the person, not just the body's chemistry, it is extraordinary and need not be applied . . . The 1980 Declaration on Euthanasia is the Church's official pronouncement that to-day we have to protect life against the dangers of technological abuse which threaten its sanctity.[38]

American cases

Decisions in the United States are deeply concerned with constitutional rights and are likely to conflict to some degree due to the different life styles to be found in, say, New England and California. They are, nevertheless, of significance to the British reader insofar as they show a trend which is becoming progressively more sympathetic to the concept of good medical practice as an arbiter of controversial life and death decisions.

The most important case in this area—although by no means the first[39]—was *Re Quinlan* in 1976[40] which concerned a 22-year-old woman who was comatose, probably as a result of a drug overdose. She was maintained on a ventilator. The hospital authorities, possibly concerned with the chance of future litigation, contended that removing her from intensive care was contrary to their professional principles, while her parents believed that the best course for her was the termination of treatment and, as everyone supposed at the time, death. The judge of first instance considered he could not substitute his judgment for that of the physicians in charge. This decision was based largely on his understanding that the patient had never previously expressed her attitudes to death other than in conversation and could not now do so. He also appointed a guardian *ad litem* for the purpose of denying a right of action to the patient's father. As judged by a rather imprecise interview with the judge concerned,[41] this opinion gave maximal regard to the patient's constitutional right to privacy—that being a right which could not be exercised by her parents. To authorise discontinuance would, in Muir J's opinion, constitute judicial approval of a forbidden act of homicide. The Supreme Court of New Jersey overturned this ruling through the classic dictum of Hughes CJ:

> We think that the State's interest *contra* weakens and an individual's right to privacy grows as the degree of bodily invasion increases and the prognosis dims. Ultimately, there comes a point at which the individual's rights overcome the State interest.[42]

The Court concluded that the only practical way to prevent destruction of those patient's rights was to allow her family to render their best judgment as to how she would exercise them in the circumstances. Following this, the court took what, initially, seems to be the unusual course of leaving the ultimate decision to the Hospital Ethics Committee. I have used the word 'unusual' in a strictly British sense in that ethical committees in the United Kingdom are set up for the sole purpose of protecting the interests of patients in the course of research and medical experimentation.[43] Similar committees in the United States are used more as 'medical review' or 'prognosis' committees.[44] They may be seen by some as having a dual function—to represent the patient but also to relieve doctors of any civil or criminal responsibility for their actions.

It will be noted later that there has been a wave of support for the use of ethical committees in preference to recourse to courts.[45]

The importance placed in the United States on a declaration of intention in the event of incapacitation is further shown in the important cases in 1981 of *Eichner* and *Storar*.[46] The New York Court of Appeals took these two cases together. Briefly, *Eichner* concerned the case of an 83-year-old seminarist, Fox, who sustained brain damage and became respirator dependent following cardiac arrest. His guardian, Father Eichner, sought authority to discontinue treatment and this right was upheld by the Supreme Court of New York on the basis that Brother Fox had expressed consistent views in life although only verbally. On appeal by the District Attorney, the Appelate Division confirmed the patient's rights in both common and constitutional law but insisted that it was the function of the court to apply a 'substituted judgment' test.[47] The important role of the 'hospital review committee' was reaffirmed but it was laid down that all such cases should be brought before a probate court to allow the State to call in its own experts. *Storar* was a rather different case of a 53-year-old incompetent with bladder cancer who required treatment by multiple blood transfusions. His mother attempted to withdraw permission for further transfusions but this was resisted by the hospital authorities. Both the Supreme Court and the Appellate Division held that the transfusions constituted 'extraordinary care' and confirmed the mother's rights as guardian.

The Court of Appeals considered that, as a matter of common law, the removal of mechanical support was proper in *Eichner's* case. The Court then distinguished *Storar* on the grounds that, since the patient, Storar, had never been competent, he had never been able to express his wishes; even if the transfusions could not cure his cancer, they could alleviate his anaemia and it was wrong to suppose that he would have chosen the negative course. A reviewer of this judgment[48] has pointed out that the majority of cases will concern *unadjudicated incompetents* to which *Storar* does not apply; nor did the Presidential Committee headed by Professor Capron[49] generalise in this area and the issue of the incompetent and uncommitted patient remained unsettled.

The problem however, was, met squarely in 1983 in the case of *Colyer*[50] where, faced with the choice between reliance on a hospital committee or on universal judicial intervention, as was said to be required in another influential case—*Saikewicz* in 1977[51]—the Court, with one dissenting opinion, came down in favour of the hospital and then preferred the use of prognosis boards rather than ethics committees. The former consist of physicians only and it would seem to be a matter of good sense that medical problems should be resolved by medical opinion. A further distinction was made regarding reference of cases to the court—such reference would not be needed if the treatment in question was merely life sustaining as opposed to life prolonging. The move away from routine court intervention has continued and was upheld in the appeal of Barber and Nejdl (see p.28). Further, even the mandatory reference of cases to ethical committees is now subject to consideration. It has been said that the sole requirement for doctors to remain within the law is that of good faith.[52] The position is, thus, approaching that in the United Kingdom—a move which is greatly welcomed by the American medical profession.[53]

Any such trend, however, is still strongly associated with, and dependent upon, existing legislation, and on a prior and firm expression of preference. This may be made through the medium of what is curiously known as 'the living will'—a process somewhat similar to carrying an organ donor card, which states, for example, 'I do not wish to be resuscitated in the event that I have been anoxic so long as to sustain severe brain damage'. The implementation of a patient's wishes may now be supported by a durable power of attorney by which the patient's agent is empowered to continue to act when the person appointing that agent becomes incapacitated.[54]

In addition, most of the United States have now introduced some form of 'Allowing to Die Act'[55] but such statutes are not free from criticism. While they may well be intended to allow patients—and, hence, their physicians—to lay down a quality of life standard, it is arguable that their main object is to protect doctors from all possibility of civil or criminal suits. Many of the enactments are fenced around with this in view. Thus, the California Natural Death Act 1976 expressly states that, in considering the implications of a longstanding 'living will', the physician may also take into account other information from the family, etc. in deciding 'whether the totality of circumstances known to the physician justify effectuating the direction'. The Act also specifically limits its application to terminal illness. It has, indeed, been suggested that 'allowing to die' legislation positively undermines the autonomy of the patient and that, at its worst, it may be a smoke screen for inadequate standards of care.[56] It could be that the status of the average incompetent is scarcely improved as a result.

It may also be that doctors are, themselves, limited by legislation in that they may be particularly vulnerable if they then appear to step out of line. True, it has been stated that, until recently, only two doctors in the United States have been tried for 'mercy killing' and, despite poor defences, both were acquitted.[57] But some of the remarks made during the course of the trials of doctors Barber and Nejdl in 1983[58] vividly illustrate the difficulties likely to arise when the law tries its hand at clinical medicine. In dismissing charges of murder and of conspiracy to commit murder at the preliminary hearing, the magistrate said:

    . . . if termination of heroic support . . . of a severely comatose
    patient is a crime, then obviously . . . one *never* hooks up patients to
    heroic support . . . One who is not connected to such equipment

can never be disconnected. Obviously it would be counter-produc-
tive to medical science to put the medical profession on such
notice.

This seems clear enough until we read that he continued: *

this conclusion does not necessarily give comfort to the medical
community in future similar decision-making processes. A decision
in this case adverse to the prosecution in no way precludes [a]
prosecutor . . . from filing similar charges when unlawful conduct
can be shown clearly and simply.[59]

The ultimate dismissal of the case was especially satisfactory considering
that the actions which were the subject of the charge accurately reflected
the published views of both the local medical and bar associations as to
what constituted good medical practice.

The situation in the United States regarding the acceptance of brain
stem death, although not uniform, seems rather less complicated. By and
large, US criminal courts have been in line with British in refusing to
admit a plea of *novus actus interveniens* when ventilator support is properly removed following assaults.[60] There are, in addition, a number of
civil cases such as *Tucker v Lower*;[61] the jury in this case refused to find
liable doctors who were sued for wrongful death having removed the
kidneys of a 'brain stem dead' man in the conditions of a 'beating heart
donor'.

Over twenty-six States have enacted statutes defining death in terms
of brain stem function in an attempt to settle any conflicting judicial
decisions. These statutes differ in content and in style.[62] The model Bill
proposed by the American Medical Association in 1979 avoids many of
the possible pitfalls:

A physician, in the exercise of his professional judgment, may
declare an individual dead in accordance with accepted medical
standards. Such declaration may be based solely on an irreversible
cessation of brain function . . .[63]

but the difficulties in drafting are considerable

6. The Neonate

Acute problems of life and death decision-making are perhaps commonest in the neonatal period.[1] In the majority of circumstances so far discussed, conditions have, in general, been slow running, allowing time for reflection. Birth, however, is an explosive moment. Moreover, because of greatly improved modern ante-natal care, and because abortion on the grounds of fetal abnormality is now available, an abnormal newborn must come as a great shock to mothers and doctors alike. Decisions concerning treatment of a defective newborn must, therefore, be taken hurriedly and in an atmosphere of high emotional tension.

The neonate's situation differs in many ways from that of the child or adult. The newborn baby cannot speak for itself; we have no yardstick by which to measure a deterioration on his or her quality of life and prognosis is not for the short term but may be needed for and expected to cover many years of life. Whoever speaks for the baby will, to a large extent, be speaking in ignorance; more importantly, whoever stands proxy, be it the parents or the State, is constrained by personal interests which may be financial, economic or emotional. The most vulnerable form of human life is utterly dependent upon surrogates who cannot be wholly objective. Small wonder that there is public anxiety.

The distasteful fact has to be faced that there are quite tenable arguments in favour of eliminating imperfect and unwanted infants—in fact, the practice was positively adopted in many earlier civilisations and persists, today, in some societies.[2] Pressure is mounting for its wider acceptance and this is based on two main precepts. The first is the growing concept of 'personhood' which can be summed up as holding that, to qualify as a person, there must be self-consciousness, self-control and a sense of past and future.[3] On these premises, the neonate is not a person and has no personal rights. Khuse and Singer in 1985, while modifying this extreme view, say: 'to allow infanticide before the onset of self-awareness cannot threaten anyone who is in a position to worry about it'[4]—which must give the neonate little confidence in those available to plead its cause.

Of more practical importance is what might be called the 'knock on' effect of the Abortion Act 1967 insofar as it is easy to see the killing of the defective neonate—or neonaticide[5]—as a catchment for a missed abortion. If we would have aborted a fetus had a chromosomal analysis been performed *in utero* and been found to be abnormal, why should we not destroy the neonate who has escaped the net? In so thinking, we are edging towards a very slippery slope[6] and there are other, more subtle, arguments designed to provide impetus. Currently, for example, it is possible to diagnose the fact of neural tube defect by amniocentesis but not the degree of abnormality suffered. Rather than abort all infants when a raised alpha-fetoprotein is discovered, would it not be more logical to wait until birth and then destroy those found to have major defects? And, in general, if it is considered dangerous to the mother to abort a fetus discovered to be abnormal after the twenty-eighth week of pregnancy, should we not simply induce labour at the most appropriate moment and kill the resulting infant?

One can argue from the reverse aspect. A pregnant woman says her mental health will be damaged if she has to support a baby and, accordingly, she may be recommended for a legal abortion. But it is well known that one of the psychiatric traumas of abortion results from a change of heart after the event. Is there not a case for allowing her to have the baby and to do away with it if she finds she still so wishes? Similar examples could be multiplied until it becomes horribly clear that neonaticide is, scientifically speaking, preferable to abortion. Good economic arguments can also be raised. Certainly, neonaticide will relieve the defective child's parents of much hardship; the State can contend—and in so doing may attract powerful support[7]—that the upkeep of the defective child is likely to be expensive and that its treatment will have an adverse effect on already stretched health resources. More sinister, the State may positively seek the consequent restriction within the community of adverse genetic conditions of both monogenic and multifactorial type.

These essentially pragmatic approaches also have their philosophical supporters. Joseph Fletcher[8], arguing from the premise that abortion serves to rid us of genetic disease, contends that the means adopted to attain a justifiable end are immaterial: 'it is only the end which makes sense of what we do'. Glover[9] has reached a similar conclusion by a contrasting route: if the main argument against abortion is that it deprives the world of a worthwhile life, then contraception, abortion and 'infanticide' are all on the same level of wrong-doing in cases where there is the same expectation of a normal child.

There are, of course, opposing views. John Fletcher has suggested that the value afforded to the infant is of a different order to that given to the fetus. He bases this on the independence of the infant, on its availability for treatment and on the development of parental acceptance of their offspring after birth. He also attacks the 'brutalisation' of those who practise euthanasia and the potential destructive social consequences of doctors turning from full care to euthanasia of the defective child.[10] The latter point is closer to the less philosophical but more instinctive abhorence which most people would have of regarding neonaticide as a legitimate extension of legal abortion. Kuhse and Singer base part of their contrary argument on the mores of communities living in the Canadian Arctic—who are said to expose unwanted female infants in the snow—and those in the Kalahari Desert, who use infanticide as a form of family planning in a nomadic existence. Such examples are unconvincing. We live in a highly developed society in which the protection of the weak, and those in need, takes an important place. Most of us would see the newborn infant—even one which is defective— as a fellow human who needs our protection and sympathy. If needs be, one can look to the law—for the law regards an infant who has achieved a separate existence as a creature in being who is entitled to its protection.

All of which seems a straightforward solution until we realise that there _are_ some infants whose quality of life is prospectively so awful that they ought not to live—infants who would have died in the past irrespective of medical care but who might, today, be maintained by using modern technology. The ensuing questions which must be addressed are, firstly, have we, in the light of the particular conditions of the neonatal period, any special mandate either to hold to or to depart from an approach which upholds the sanctity of life? Secondly, if we reject that approach on the grounds of special need, how far are we to go along the quality of life road? The answers are not easy. We have moved from the simple doctor/patient relationship and must now involve a third party— the parents—in any discussion. The rights of all three must be considered within clinical, moral and legal contexts.

The clinical problem

Excluding disasters such as giving drugs to a pregnant woman which are toxic or teratogenic to the fetus, congenital disease may be looked upon as having four major origins—monogenetic, multifactorial genetic, environmental or chromosomal disorders. It would be unrealistic to embark on a full consideration of these processes within the conceptual limitations of this book,[11] but the following brief summary attempts to set the scene for the purposes of the present debate, and for that of the abortion issue which is considered in the next chapter.

Monogenetic disease can be attributed to a specific gene; the method of inheritance is, thus, understood and its occurrence is predictable mathematically. In such an instance, the genetic counsellor has hard facts on which to work and specific defects to search for during antenatal care. Monogenetic disease may be sex-linked and then, with rare exceptions, is transmitted by the female but is manifested in the male. Perhaps the best known example of this is haemophilia. While the science of genetic engineering—or better, of recombinant DNA technology—is improving rapidly, it is, at present, fair to say that not all monogenetic disease can be identified _in utero_, and that it may be impossible to determine its presence early in pregnancy—although this problem may be solved by the development of chorionic villus sampling.

Multifactorial disease derives from a combination of genetic and environmental sources. Either can be the predominant factor and the effect is capricious both in the occurrence and in the quality of the defect. Genetic sources can only be predicted empirically, while environmental sources are often unassessable, although improvements in techniques, such as the extending horizons of ultrasonography, are changing the face of obstetric practice. Nevertheless, the defects which are diagnosable at birth are physical and, consequently, potentially treatable; neural tube defect is the most important of such conditions for our purpose here. Environmental disease is exemplified by viral infection in the mother—of which German measles is pre-eminent—by rhesus immunisation or by drug therapy or abuse. The medico-legal significance of such conditions is that they are, in general, preventable.

Chromosomal disease may be due to changes in the structure of chromosomes or in their number. The primary occurence of the former is random—although some conditions, such as exposure to ionising radiation, increase the possibility of change. A change in the number of chromosomes is, similarly, unforeseeable but the incidence of abnormality increases with maternal age, and this indicates to the obstetrician a group of mothers who are at special risk. Numerical chromosomal abnormalities which are compatible with the development of the fetus to full term are of the 'trisomy' type—i.e. particular chromosomes are present as a triplet rather than as a normal pair. Many such trisomies provoke such extreme abnormality as to be incompatible with life beyond the neonatal stage, others, particularly those associated with the sex chromosomes, may result in a comparatively normal, although sexually underdeveloped child.

The common feature of chromosomal disorders is a degree of mental defect; this can neither be treated nor quantified at birth. At the same time, some additional physical defect is likely to be present, but this, is usually correctable. Down's syndrome, or mongolism, is the most common form of trisomy apart from those which affect the sex chromosomes. While it is perhaps obvious, it is pointed out that, quite apart from congenital defect, a severely defective neonate may also result from injury sustained during birth. A major distinction between such cases and those caused by congenital disease lies in the fact that antenatal care need not have indicated a valid reason for specific management, including abortion, in the birth-injury cases. It follows that there is something of a hard core of cases of spastic paralysis associated with mental disability which will not be eliminated by genetic counselling.

Clinical attitudes to neonatal defects are liable to polarisation. On the one hand, the sanctity of life proponents—or 'vitalists'—will say that all defects should be treated at all costs in an effort to maintain life; on the other, perfectionists may argue that it is our duty to eliminate genetic disease whatever its gravity, since both genetic and chromosomal abnormality, once introduced into the family, will persist in future generations. As always, neither extreme is wholly tenable. A compromise is essential and this finds expression in the principle of selective non-treatment of the newborn. Any such policy is open to the criticism that it fails

> to give any idea of just when an infant becomes a candidate for non-treatment or merely palliative care . . . we are never told just what the handicaps are or what the criteria are that distinguish those infants whose parents should be allowed to discontinue care from those whose parents who should not have any such request honoured.[12]

For ease of description, I intend to consider this proposition from the point of view only of neural defects and Down's syndrome. To understand the nature of these conditions is to avoid many of the conceptual errors which have come to be associated with the management of the defective newborn.

Neural tube defects

These conditions may range from the virtual absence of the brain (anencephaly), which is inconsistent with life, to comparatively minor residual musculo-skeletal dysfunction, with or without some intellectual impairment, following treatment. The essential features of the *severe* neural tube defect are, firstly, that it is likely to be fatal in the absence of treatment and, secondly, that, in many instances, treatment may be painful and eventually unsatisfactory. In the worst event, the child may survive as a virtual ament but with sufficient cerebral function to appreciate pain and discomfort.

It is within this group of infants particularly that the policy of selective non-treatment has developed. The underlying philosophy is that it is the doctor's responsibility not to: 'prolong . . . suffering unnecessarily . . . in an infant whose chance for acceptable growth and development is negligible'.[13] Major credit for the scientific development of the regimen must be attributed to Lorber who, it is worth noting, was moved to his policy by the results of his earlier commitment to compulsive treatment.[14] The basis for this motivation lies in an attempt to promote the best interests of the child. It is clear that this principle is difficult to apply in this context because an assessment of what is best is being made by adults; in practice, it can only mean that the outcome is decided on the understanding that the interests of others involved are subjugated to those of the infant.

Lorber's approach, which has been used world-wide as a template for decison-making, has been to define the criteria which indicate a poor prognosis and, having recognised these in a neonate, to recommend against operative treatment;[15] he thus avoids the general charge of vagueness which has been noted above. A typical consequence of such policy has been that forty-nine out of seventy-one untreated children survived for less than two months and only two were alive after one year. By contrast, eighty-six per cent of treated children survived, only twenty-three per cent having residual handicap. Two features need stressing. First, this is a classic example of applying the productive/non-productive treatment test. Not only would a high proportion of the untreated cases have died despite heroic effort but, also, there is no obligation to subject a patient to repetitive pain in order to achieve a life of chronic suffering.[16] Secondly, selective non-treatment is as equivalent to passive euthanasia in the newborn as it is in the adult. The same questions arise as to whether this approach is preferable to active intervention and the problem will be reverted to later.

The Down's syndrome baby

By contrast to those infants with severe physical defect, the uncomplicated Down's syndrome baby has no intention of dying. If it is to do so, it must be helped on its way and this implies either active intervention or the withholding of such basic support as feeding. There can be no selective non-treatment because there is no treatment to give, and the intended death of the baby can only be categorised as neonaticide.

Moreover, while we all know what pain and immobility are, in this instance we have nothing by which to judge the infant's quality of life because the Down's syndrome infant himself knows of no alternative; the child is not going to complain about his condition, and it follows that anyone who does so on his behalf is arrogating an ill-founded right to do so. For this reason, I would disagree with Williams who wrote:

> If a wicked fairy told me she was about to transform me into a Down's baby and asked if I would prefer to die, I should certainly answer yes.[17]

That is not what the baby is being asked. For all we know, the Down's syndrome infant is perfectly contented in his own inner world. An infant which has been born alive has rights of its own[18] and to bring about the death of a baby simply because of its abnormal chromosomal and hence its subnormal mental-state is dangerously close to genetic engineering on a societal basis, or to the racial eugenics of the 1930s and 40s.

There is, thus, considerable disparity in the evaluation of the neural tube defective neonate on the one hand and of the mentally retarded on the other. The situation is, however, complicated by the fact that about a quarter of Down's syndrome infants also have physical defects that are incompatible with life if they are left untreated. But, again in contrast to severe spina bifida, many of the treatments required are relatively simple in the hands of today's paediatric surgeons and they generally subject the infant to the stresses no worse than those of a standard intra-abdominal or intra-thoracic operation. Such cases present something of a half-way house in therapeutic decision-making but the essential underlying thread is that to refuse an operation to a Down's baby which would be provided without hesitation for a mentally normal patient is to make a social rather than a medical decision. The best interests of the patient have then become a secondary feature. [19]

The legal position

The attitude of the law in the United Kingdom to selective non-treatment of physical defect has never been tested in the courts. The nearest approach was the affair of *Stephen Quinn*[20] in 1981 in which a surgeon was reported to the police for supposedly refusing to sustain a baby with spina bifida. In the event, the Director of Public Prosecutions decided to take no action.

It seems reasonable to assume that this would always be the case in the absence of malicious intent or of reckless disregard for either parental or peer opinion. Practice of this particular form of passive euthanasia has been openly reported in medical literature and has been duplicated in many countries. There is little doubt that it qualifies as good medical practice. The words of Farquharson J sum up what is likely to be the general judicial view, although it will be clear that I do not agree with the assumption as it was applied in the particular circumstances of *Arthur* (see below p.70). The judge said:

> I imagine you will think long and hard before deciding that eminent doctors have evolved standards that amount to committing a crime. [21]

Quite what such standards ought to be and how they should be uniformly applied is a matter for debate. Perhaps it should be through the medium of wide-ranging legislation coupled with a code of practice—a somewhat similar arrangement to that which currently governs the association between brain stem death and the transplantation of organs. The matter is discussed in greater detail at p.115.

While the management of severe physical defect is, thus, reasonably well agreed, there is far less medical consensus as to that of infants born suffering from Down's syndrome, and this is particularly apparent when the condition is complicated by physical defect. Here we can look to reported court decisions.

British cases

The most important British case is that of *In re B*[22] in 1981. The infant concerned was born with Down's syndrome and suffered from the fairly common complication of duodenal atresia; the treatment of this condition is not overly difficult but death is inevitable in the absence of surgery. B's parents refused permission for the operation and the surgeons took the somewhat unusual step of asking the local authority to apply for court wardship. The court first gave permission for treatment, but the doctors to whom the baby was referred refused to act in the absence of parental consent, whereupon Ewbank J rescinded the order. The local authority, having discovered other surgeons willing to act, appealed, and the Court of Appeal ordered that the operation be performed.

The issue here was decided on the 'best interests' of the child. The parents contended that, since no one could tell what the life of a mongol child would be like, it would be in the child's interests not to have the operation; the local authority considered that good adoptive arrangements could be made so that the child would have a relatively happy life for twenty to thirty years. [23]

Templeman LJ's judgment included the following rhetorical question:

. . . was the child's life going to be so demonstrably awful that it should be condemned to die or was the kind of life so imponderable that it would be wrong to condemn her to die?

The court concluded that it was wrong that life should be terminated because she had another disability in addition to being a mongol and, significantly, that:

she should be put in the same position as *any other mongol child* (my emphasis) and must be given the chance to live an existence. [24]

Three months later came a second case which, being taken in the criminal court, attracted far more public notice.

R v Arthur[25]

In this unique, although, surprisingly, not officially reported case, Dr Arthur, a physician of undisputed skill and integrity, made the following observation in the notes of a new-born baby suffering from apparently uncomplicated Down's syndrome: 'Parents do not wish it to survive. Nursing care only.' He also prescribed large doses of the drug dihydrocodein which was intended to suppress the child's desire for food. The infant died some sixty-nine hours after birth. Following post-mortem examination, death was ascribed to 'multilobular pneumonia due to lung stasis due to dihydrocodein poisoning in an infant with Down's syndrome'. [26] Dr Arthur was then charged with murder.

During the trial, the defence adduced evidence to the effect that the infant had abnormalities of the heart, lungs and brain. Despite the fact that the same defence pathologist, acting in concert with the pathologist for the Crown, had originally signed a report ignoring such abnormalities, [26] and despite the fact that the Crown pathologist's opinion was not markedly altered by his colleague's change of opinion, the charge of murder was then withdrawn and one of attempted murder was substituted. Dr Arthur was found not guilty of this lesser offence.

There are both positive and negative specific points to be derived from *Arthur*. On the negative side, I believe the case to be irrelevant as to defining the law. [27] Murder, in the popular sense of the word, was the one thing of which Dr Arthur was certainly innocent. It was always inconceivable that a jury would find him so guilty and I submit that the decision to charge with murder was ill-judged. In the circumstances, Dr Arthur was at risk of a mandatory life sentence[28] and he was, therefore, forced to defend himself rather than his principles. His line of defence, although perfectly valid, was specific to the circumstances of the case and was, in the opinion of many, not conducive to establishing scientific truth.[29] Dr Arthur might, however, have been guilty of manslaughter or even of a very much lesser offence under the Children and Young Persons Act 1933, s.1. The nature of the trial precluded assessment of these possibilities.

The positive lesson from the case is that the traditional reluctance of a jury and of the judiciary to convict a doctor of criminality in relation to patient care was upheld and, to my mind, the significance of the trial is limited to this conclusion. Kennedy's view that its importance goes deeper is discussed below (p.68). One can only speculate on what would have happened had the child been perfectly normal. Brahams[30] has suggested that the jury would probably have acquitted even if the infant had survived for fourteen days, but she thought that this would have been scarcely reasonable. While agreeing with this, I still believe that neither the length of survival nor the physical state of the victim should have been material to an attempt. It has been thought that the trial of Dr Arthur is best forgotten; at the same time, it has been pointed out that the eminent medical men who gave evidence presumably still hold the opinions they expressed and that these may, accordingly, have gained further currency within the medical profession.[31] The case, therefore, still has to be considered in some depth.

The general implications of Arthur

It has been said that there are surprisingly few substantive issues in medical ethics that the Arthur case does not raise.[32] There will be wide agreement with this view but, for the present, I intend to confine discussion to the practical issue of where the law stands. A good starting proposition is that the case decided that a joint decision by doctors and parents to let a baby die is not unlawful.[33] To examine this, it is useful to take both of the relevant cases together—despite the fact that In re B does not seem to have been referred to in Arthur. First we must examine the 'rights' of the various parties.

The rights of the parents

The precise wording of Dr Arthur's case notes—'parents do not wish it to survive. Nursing care only'—implies an understanding that compelling authority is vested in the parents; certainly, decisions will be reached as a result of discussions but, in the end, it is the parents who will or will not consent to the form of medical management of their infant. It is not difficult to find support for such an interpretation. To take but one

example each from the British legal and medical professions:
> There is a strong argument for keeping the law out of these cases . . .
> the decision of the parents should prevail

said Williams;[34] and the *British Medical Journal* backed this with:
> in the absence of a clear code to which society adheres there is no
> justification for usurping parents' rights.[35]

But what are these 'rights' that are held to be so imperative? The status
of the fetus vis-à-vis its mother is discussed in the next chapter. For
present purposes, it needs only to be noted that it attains a right not to be
killed after the twenty-eighth week of gestation—a right which is subject
only to its mother's superior right to life. There is no danger to the
mother after parturition and it should follow logically that the neonate
has an absolute right to life,—given an assumption of self-ownership,
there is no morally permissible infanticide [used in its non-statutory
sense] or destruction of a viable fetus'.[36] It has also already been noted
that an infant having an independent existence has legal rights of its
own.[37] Thus far, no solid case can be made for any parental rights to
neonaticide.

Nevertheless, in the absence of understanding on the part of the child,
the principle of parental jurisdiction is well established as to consent to
medical treatment[38] and this, presumably, is what justifies the *British
Medical Journal* in advising: 'All patients . . . have a right to accept or
reject medical treatment . . . As the infant cannot take a decision
personally it is the responsibility of the parents to take the decision'.[39]
But the Family Law Reform Act 1969, s.8 covers parental consent only
when the decisions made are to the child's advantage. Can we honestly
say that the parents can and should decide that their child must die when
there is no evidence that this is its preferred option? The implausibility
of contending that this is so becomes clear once we remove the case from
the hospital setting. What would be the public reaction were the parents
of a child born at home to allow it to die by neglect simply because they
'did not wish it to survive'? It would surely be seen as murder.[40] Or, given
these parental powers, why should a similar attitude not be adopted
towards an older child who has sustained cerebral or spinal injury in the
playground? Parents cannot simply withdraw their parental responsibili-
ties[41] and there is world-wide legislation which is specifically designed to
prevent parents harming their children. It becomes increasingly difficult
to see why they should be seen as excused for doing so in the neonatal
stage.

Ayer, a philosopher who supports the quality of life doctrine, drew
attention to thalidomide babies and to the fact that many of them have
developed into reasonably happy children. He continued:
> A great deal depends here on the attitude of the parents. I am
> inclined to say that the child should be allowed to live if the parents
> are resolved to care for it lovingly.[42]

Such a conclusion virtually eliminates the interest of the child as a significant factor in the equation and takes no note of any contrary view of parental decision-making. 'Parents are bad decision makers',[43] it has been said, and this is particularly so when decisions are taken at a time of maximum emotional stress. One cannot simply ignore such emphatic views as:

> Reliance on the parents' judgment allows for the worst and most arbitrary factors to determine which infant lives or dies.[44]

The infant's rights

The rights of the infant in any management decision derive unarguably from the facts which have already been outlined—that, once having attained a separate existence, the child is an independent being, and that this is so despite the fact that it is restricted by being unable to express its wishes without assistance. It follows that the only principle on which proxy decisions can properly be made is that of the neonate's best interests. In particular, a 'substituted judgment test' is inappropriate because, as was pointed out in the introduction to this chapter, there is no previous experience on which to draw and because the interests of those making the judgment may compete with those of the infant.[45]

It has been suggested that the infant's independent status carries with it both rights to death and rights to life which are comparable to those of the adult.[46] But, despite its logicality, it would seem that the former premise is, at least, uncertain. A fetal right to death has been consistently denied and this was confirmed in the case of McKay,[47] the major British case in which an action for 'wrongful life' on the part of the fetus was expressly excluded. Extrapolation from the fetus to the neonate is not easy because of the all-important intervening assumption of a separate existence. Nevertheless, it is difficult to see how there can be any right to neonatal death because of being born with some devastating (but not life-threatening) defect if there is no such legal entity as a 'wrongful life'. Practical conditions, in any event, prohibit the neonate from adopting the adult option of suicide. The issue central to the post-Arthur debate is whether or not non-voluntary euthanasia can be rightly substituted.

On the other hand, the neonate, as an independent being, certainly has a right to treatment and, in the event of physical defect, it may demand that treatment on the basis of a productive/non-productive treatment test, the overriding feature of which would be the relative pain and suffering involved.[48] But it is stretching semantics too far to suggest that to die is in the best interests of a child who is neither in pain nor, apparently, unhappy. It is also worth noting that the mentally retarded but otherwise physically normal neonate is simply not considered as a candidate for the category of 'severely defective' in the United States.[49] The mental state of the neonate is, in short, something which affects society rather than the subject. The acceptance of this is implicit in the words of the Court of Appeal in *In re B*:

> The judge of first instance erred in considering the wishes of the parents rather than the best interests of the child.

Once that view is accepted, the treatment of the common physical complications of Down's syndrome is clarified. The test becomes one of feasibility: if life-saving surgery is feasible for the 'normal' infant, it cannot morally be withheld from one whose disability consists of being unable to measure up to society's standards of a normal intelligence. And while this approach may appear to be unduly academic and divorced from the rigours of the real world, it has the practical merit of avoiding uncertainties and inconsistencies in prognosis.[50]

Squaring the circle

What, then, is the conclusion to be drawn from the British cases and on what evidence is that to be based? Williams provides a good starting point when he indicates that the court would *not* have ordered an operation in *In re B* had the child been likely to suffer in life and, from this, extrapolates that parents and doctors are *entitled* to decide against a life-saving operation when there is positive evidence that such a 'life of suffering' is probable.[51] But the entitlement is certainly not absolute and must be child-orientated. Otherwise, it would be justifiable for parents to reject a normal child, which, clearly, they cannot do.[52] It is murder for a parent to withhold food and water from a child so that it dies, and that must apply irrespective of the child's prospective mental status. The words in *In re B*: 'She should be put in the same position as any other mongol child' indicate that the court would not have entertained the idea of non-treatment of a physically healthy mongol in whom non-treatment must mean non-feeding; the impression given is that this possibility never entered the judges' minds.

The most positive and most recent evidence on the point to come from a Commonwealth court is to be found in the opinion of Vincent J in the 1986 Australian case of F v F:[53]

> No parent, no doctor, no court has any power to determine whether the life of any child, however disabled that child may be, will be deliberately taken from it . . . [the law] does not permit decisions to be made concerning the quality of life nor does it enable any assessment to be made as to the value of any human being.

Clear as that may be in Australia, it is still difficult in Britain to equate *In re B*, which was a case concerned with simple treatment and is the case which I maintain represents the definitive law in this field, with the later case of *Arthur* which involved the far more controversial issue of feeding. Legal thinking in the area is not easy to follow. Williams, for example, says at one point:

> It must be recognised that a parent who withholds nourishment in order to cause an infant to die is in the same moral position as if he

had killed by positive act and general public opinion would not
accept the killing of infants on account of defect.[54]

In a companion article, he concludes:

It seems clear on principle that anything done to a baby against the
known wishes of the parents is prima facie an assault . . . The
consent of parents even extends to feeding.[55]

Yet again, he says:

It is too positive a view as to the present state of the law that doctors
and parents can legally agree to allow a handicapped baby to die
provided that no-one challenges their decisions at the time . . . The
criminal law should stay its hand.[56]

Kennedy considered the current legal situation to be in a mess but,
nevertheless, believed that *Arthur* made new law with the effect that it is
now lawful to treat a baby with sedating drugs and to offer no further care
by way of food or drugs or surgery if certain criteria are met.[57] These are,
said Kennedy:

First that the child must be irreversibly disabled and, secondly,
rejected by its parents . . . The judge drew a distinction between
sedating the baby and passively letting it die and doing a positive act
to kill the baby, for example, giving it a death dealing dose of drugs.
The latter, he said, would be unlawful, the former lawful.

If this is the law, then I submit that it is bad law. I certainly agree that
there is a major emotional difference between the two processes. But
allowing a baby to waste away is manifestly unkind; the effect on the
baby—and on the nurses and other attendants—is likely to be more
traumatic than is a single positive lethal act.[58] If this latter, more
'humane' method is illegal—and no doctor is likely to adopt it—then the
logical conclusion is that the more 'inhumane' should be, at least,
equally illegal.[59] I believe that this must be the conclusion to be drawn
from *In re B*, and it is stretching interpretation too far to suggest that it is
overturned by *Arthur*. Brahams[60] has put it more succinctly in that,
insofar as *Arthur* conflicts with the Court of Appeal decision in *In re B*, it
is a jury decision from an inferior court which would seem to be inconsistent and is, therefore, wrong.

There is authoritative evidence to support this view. After the *Arthur*
trial, the Attorney General said:

I am satisfied that the law relating to murder and to attempted
murder is the same now as it was before the trial . . . and that it is the
same irrespective of the wishes of the parents or any other person
having a duty to care for the victim.[61]

Earlier, Brahams concluded from the *Arthur* case that either the law
was out of step or it had evolved double standards to the specific
advantage of doctors.[62] There is, indeed, some indication that there is a
measure of general acceptance to the effect that, whereas parents acting
alone to accomplish their baby's death would be guilty of an offence, they

would be exonerated if they were working in concert with their doctors —in practice, the effect of such interplay would be to transfer the onus subtly to the doctor whom the law is either unwilling or unable to prosecute.

Is it, in fact, unable to do so? The question hinges not so much on any supposed differences between commission and omission but on the nature of the duty of care which the doctor owes to the neonatal patient.

The question of the duty of care has already been discussed broadly in relation to the adult (p.50) and it would seem that the argument in favour of such a relationship is not so much diminished but rather positively augmented in the case of the incompetent noenate. In the absence of breast feeding, a newborn has no one to turn to for sustenance other than the doctor. Distinctions which can be made between an authority to act and a duty to act cease to be relevant in such circumstances.[63] The simpler view would surely be that of Brahams[64] who said that, while the criminal law does not impose obligations on a person to care for another, nonetheless, when care is assumed, so also is responsibility for both acts and omissions. By being in charge of a ward, the doctor assumes responsibility for all those in that ward—if he does not, then the phrase 'in charge' is meaningless. That being so, non-feasance may possibly suffice for murder[65] and the *British Medical Journal* has conceded that there may be room for charges based on omission when a duty of care exists.[66] The doctrine of 'double effect' cannot be invoked on either clinical or moral grounds and any suggestion that infant feeding constitutes extraordinary or non-productive treatment is grotesque.

The possible alternatives to doctor/parent decision making concerning selective non-treatment are, effectively, reduced to the use of ethical committees of the type which is so popular in the United States, or to recourse to wardship proceedings. The former has little professional support in the United Kingdom[67] and the latter attracted considerable criticism in the wake of both *In re B* and *Arthur*. Williams, for example, said:

> . . . the judges should not use the wardship procedure to supplant the parents[68]

and there was much newspaper criticism, including a cynical assessment of the cost of B's survival at £100000.[69] The Secretary of the British Medical Association said of the *Arthur* case:

> It is a crushing indictment of our legal system that men such as . . . Leonard Arthur should be subjected to criminal prosecution for carrying out with great devotion and skill, procedures which are accepted by the profession as in the best interests of patients.[70]

The Lancet[71] criticised the case in that the opportunity to secure a judgment declaring a general principle was forsaken and it will be seen when the American experience is discussed below that difficulties *are* introduced when the courts become involved in clinical decisions. But it has been pointed out that Dr Arthur's decision was an ethical one rather than clinical[72]—and concern has been expressed that, currently, the code of ethics in this field is being determined by doctors alone.[73] There is much to be said for the view that it should be for a jury, faced with a problem of lack of care and, therefore, untrammelled by the fear of imposing an undeserved long prison sentence, to demonstrate whether these are, indeed, the ethics of society. It may well be that society *is* more concerned with the well-being of the family rather than with the rights of the newborn.[74] Whether or not this is so, the attitudes of the medical profession will be very influential given the present state of the law. They merit analysis.

Doctors' attitudes

Following the decision in *In re B*, a leading article in the *British Medical Journal*[75] pointed out the illogicality of failing to treat congenital abnormalities in children simply on the grounds that they were Down's syndrome subjects. Admitting that the answer to the treatment of such infants might not always be clear, the writer counselled against 'that slippery slope that would lead to the nonchalant taking of lives found to be substandard, inconvenient or expensive'. At the same time, Professor Lorber was quoted as proposing that treatment should not be withheld if the baby was simply mentally retarded,[76] although it is difficult to see what treatment there is to withhold from such a child. The editorial commentator was clearly sympathetic to the infant's circumstances and the major criticisms expressed in subsequent correspondence were largely directed towards the possible extension of legal powers over the doctor involved in the treatment of grossly handicapped infants—thereby, again, demonstrating a failure to appreciate the unique position that the mongol, or any other mentally subnormal person, who is only minimally physically deformed occupies in the protocol of managment.

However, a change could be discerned in the Association's attitudes following *Arthur*. The immediately relevant—or 'post-*Arthur*'—leading article in the *British Medical Journal*[77] started: 'Paediatricians—and indeed all doctors—will have been relieved that Dr Leonard Arthur was acquitted of the criminal charges made against him'. The question must then arise: Relieved from what? Was the British Medical Association now less mindful of abstract principles and more concerned that the profession was under attack? That is certainly an impression which can be gained from the tone of subsequent articles[78] and the underlying reaction may account for some of the editorial conclusions which are difficult to reconcile. 'Doctors', said the leader writer, 'who believe that their management of newborn babies with severe handicaps was right in the past should not be deflected by Dr Arthur's experiences'. He then continued:

An infant with physical or mental handicaps that are not immediately life threatening should not, we believe, be allowed to die by default.

The comparison implied in the former statement is irrelevant; the latter conclusion is inconsistent with support for Dr Arthur, as several correspondents soon pointed out.[79] There is no suggestion from the information available that the infant involved was regarded as physically abnormal at the time 'nursing care only' was prescribed, and certainly none that it was in pain.[80] There is bound to be confusion within the profession until this is openly recognised. Kennedy[81] has quoted an influential television programme which showed quite clearly that, despite the wealth of expert evidence given in the trial, a substantial proportion of paediatricians would not have supported the regimen which Dr Arthur adopted. The Secretary of the British Medical Association, while at the same time deprecating the prosecution of Dr Arthur, has advocated the policy: 'If a child is not suffering from a life-threatening abnormality, the same treatment is given as is given for any other child'.[82]

The danger of uncertainty is that views may become so polarised that they inhibit compromise. There is a tendency for some elements of the British medical profession to cry 'defensive medicine' in the spirit of crying 'wolf' when their professional authority is questioned.[83] Nevertheless, almost everyone would agree that there is a real hazard that an imposed move towards an absolute sanctity of life ethos could result in the enforcement of unnecessary and unrewarding treatments on severely deformed neonates—and although he denies the inference, this might be an unfortunate consequence of Kennedy's drive towards greater societal control of medicine. It could well be, however, that the main threat lies at the other extreme of a quality of life stance. The notion of the wedge or domino effect is unpopular but its occurrence is a fact of life and particularly of life in an increasingly materialistic world. There is a danger that 'quality' of life standards may be applied with increasing refinement and that they may be set ever more subjectively. The dilemma is well expressed in a letter written in the wake of Arthur:

> The new teaching that the quality of life, as judged by other people, equals the value of that life is the greatest nonsense of all. Our profession is dedicated to caring for the sick. Its latest dogma allows discrimination against the sick.[84]

The British Medical Association originally suggested that problems of neonatal management might be resolved through peer review[85] but this does nothing to clarify the issues. Absolution through the confessional carries little weight in the secular world. More positive action is called for and the Association, in fact, issued a later categoric statement which is now official policy:

> A malformed infant has the same rights as a normal infant. It follows that ordinary non-medical care which is necessary for the

maintenance of the life of a normal infant should not be withheld
from a malformed infant[86]
and, at the time as the statement was issued, the Association's Under-
Secretary added that this meant, among other things, 'making sure that
the child was fed unless there were clinical reasons to the contrary'.[87]

Thus, there has been a definite shift within the leadership of the
profession back to the 'pre-*Arthur*' stance—a stance which is almost
certainly more acceptable to the general public.

The American experience

The American experience does much to underline the difficulties and
conflict which may arise when not only parents and doctors are in dispute
as to the management of a defective neonate but also when the judiciary
and the legislature are at loggerheads.

There has been no case comparable to that of Dr Arthur because
failure to feed an uncomplicated case of Down's syndrome would not be
regarded as a management option which is available in the United
States.[88] On the other hand, there has been more courtroom activity
associated with severe defect than there has been in Britain and, again,
there have been differences of judicial opinion.[89] In the 1970s, there was
a strong bias toward a sanctity of life ethos and a tendency to order
treatment on the basis of feasibility. It was held that the issue was not
founded on the prospective quality of life but lay, rather, between the
in-built hazards of the treatment as compared with the almost certain risk
of death if the treatment was withheld—surgery was to be performed so
long as it was needed and feasible.[90] Similarly, it was held in a later case
that: 'if there is any lifesaving treatment available, it must be undertaken
regardless of the quality of life that will result'.[91] And, in a severe case of
spina bifida, it was said that the infant's interests superseded the parental
right to withhold treatment when there was a reasonable opportunity to
live and to surmount handicaps. 'Children', said the judge, 'are not
property whose disposition is left to parental discretion without hind-
rance'.[92]

On the other hand, parental rights are jealously guarded under the
United States constitution and a marked change in attitudes seems to
have evolved with the turn of the decade. Thus, in other cases from New
England, the Juvenile Court, taking the position of the parents of an
abandoned infant, found itself empowered to decide that some types of
treatment were inappropriate;[93] and, in the well-publicised case of baby
Jane Doe, it was decided that, in refusing surgery for multiple deformi-
ties: 'the parents had elected a treatment which was within accepted
medical standards'.[94] This case was appealed and the judgment confirmed on the grounds that: 'to allow any person to by-pass the statutory
requirements would catapult him into the very heart of the family circle
to challenge the parents' responsibility to care for their children'.

The rather extraordinary 1981 case of *Phillip B*[95] concerned a twelve -year-old Down's syndrome child who had a congenital heart defect and who had been in residential care since birth. It was not, therefore, a neonatal case but it serves to demonstrate the great importance which American courts are likely to put on parental rights. Two cardiologists concurred that the child would enjoy a significant extension of life span if his defect was surgically corrected. The surgical mortality was assessed as lying between three and ten per cent but, nevertheless, both regarded the condition as correctable. The parents refused permission for operation and the matter was taken to appeal. The Court of Appeal then confirmed the dismissal of a petition that the child be declared a dependent of the Court for the purposes of treatment—this because the operation would subject him to a greater than average risk. This remarkable judgment was based on the 14th Amendment to the US Constitution which holds that legal judgments regarding the value of child-rearing patterns should be kept to a minimum so long as the child is afforded the best available opportunity to fulfil his potential in society; the State must show a serious burden of justification before abridging parental autonomy.

Such a decision is said to be inconsistent with existing jurisprudence on parental duties[96] and can be compared with the Canadian case of *Dawson*.[97] There, the parents refused replacement of a shunt in their six-year-old hydrocephalic child. McKenzie J held that: 'There looms the awful possibility that, without the shunt, the child will endure in a state of increasing disability and pain'. It followed that replacing the shunt was a necessary procedure to which the parents could not object.

It was, however, another Down's baby which precipitated what became a major medico-political crisis in the United States. The decision in that case, *Re Infant Doe*,[98] was that the value of parental autonomy outweighed the infant's right to live when a 'minimally adequate quality of life was non-existent'. This seems a remarkable assessment when the only known physical defect was an easily correctable tracheo-oesophageal fistula. As a result, the Federal Administration attempted to apply the Rehabilitation Act 1973, s.504 (which protects the rights of the handicapped) to the defective newborn but instructions to this effect from the Secretary of Health and Human Services were struck down by the United States District Court of the District of Columbia on the grounds that the section 'could never be applied blindly and without any correlation of the burdens and intrusions which might result'.[99] A similar fate then overtook revised Federal regulations, medical non-treatment being distinguished from discrimination on the grounds that the latter could only be shown when treatment for conditions other than the handicap was withheld.[100]

A need for legislation?

The American experience clearly indicated the need for clarification and, as a result, the Child Abuse Amendments of 1984 were passed to amend the Child Abuse Prevention and Treatment Act 1974.[101] These defined the term 'withholding of medically indicated treatment'. Although such action was prohibited, the amendments laid down the conditions under which failure to provide treatment for defective neonates would *not* be included under that heading. These were when:

   (a) the infant is chronically and incurably comatose
   (b) the provision of such treatment would
      (i) merely prolong dying
      (ii) not be effective in ameliorating or correcting all of the infant's life threatening conditions or
      (iii) otherwise be futile in terms of the survival of the infant and the treatment itself under such circumstances would be inhumane.

It should be noted that the provision of nutrition and hydration was considered obligatory in all circumstances.

Whether such legislation is necessary in the United Kingdom is debatable.[102] On the whole, it would seem that the situation is so confused in both professional and lay minds that an enabling Act, backed by a code of conduct might well be useful. Its possible form is discussed further in Chapter 9.

There is considerable force in Havard's arguments[103] against detailed restrictions in any legislation and the American Act could well be faulted on this point. It does not, for example, take into consideration the difficult clinical decisions involved in the care of the premature infant. Some twelve per cent of very premature infants may be expected to suffer severe disability;[104] the paediatrician is, thus, effectively taking a selective treatment decision whenever he admits a premature infant to intensive care. He does not and cannot know, however, whether an individual infant will be compromised and selection, if it is practised, can only be based on such ill-defined criteria as knowing that the prognosis worsens as the birth weight decreases. At the end of the day, the most significant balancing factor may be that of the availability of the necessary resources. It is a pity, although no doubt inevitable, that such factors must have a place in some of the most difficult decisions which are taken in medical practice.

One tenable view, however, would be that the best way to avoid problems in the management of the neonate is through improved arrangements for abortion and attention must now be given to that central subject.

7. Abortion

The history of abortion shows that the procedure has always been controversial but that disapproval has been less severe than many would expect. The moral objection rests, of course, on general condemnation of the deliberate taking of human life. It follows that the degree of such objection is governed by the extent to which the fetus is accorded the status of a human being. It would be hard to devise an anti-abortion argument if the fetus has no such status until it is born. If, however, human life begins with conception, then any form of abortion is immoral unless justified on special grounds—and so are several other practices associated with modern reproductive techniques including, for example, embryocide and displanting methods of contraception. The whole abortion controversy thus hinges on the age-old question—at what moment does human life begin? Insofar as 'life' is a continuum from conception to death, the chances of finding an answer which will satisfy everyone are remote, but it is nevertheless important to review the options briefly. Those which spring most readily to mind are: the attainment of personhood—which has already been noted and discarded—birth, viability, quickening, the appearance of a human form, the formation of nervous tissue, segmentation, implantation and conception. [1] Each will be considered in its claim for recognition.

There is great convenience in the choice of birth as a determinant of human life. In particular, it is a moment in development which is of fundamental legal importance. The question of fetal rights will be considered later. For the present, it need only be observed that any such rights do not *materialise* until the fetus is born alive and attains a separate existence—that is, has shown itself to be capable of breathing after being completely extruded from the mother. At this point the infant becomes a person in being, and is subject to the general laws of homicide and to the specific law relating to infanticide or child murder. [2]

In addition, a fundamental physiological change occurs at birth in that the infant ceases to depend upon its mother for its oxygen supply. On the other hand, a full term fetus is as well developed anatomically as is the neonate and it would be absurd to suggest that it would be both ethically and legally acceptable to kill it during the first stage of labour but wholly immoral and criminal to do so in the third stage. The Infant Life (Preservation) Act 1929 of England and Wales, which established child destruction as an offence, was introduced specifically to counter

75

any doubts on the subject (Appendix B).

The concept of viability is frequently misunderstood. It requires more of an infant than being born alive and refers to its capacity to survive after birth. The subject is confused by the wording of the Abortion Act 1967, s. 5 which refers to the Infant Life (Preservation) Act 1929 as 'protecting the life of the viable foetus'. In fact, the 1929 Act is concerned only with the fetus which is capable of being born alive. In laying down that a gestation of twenty-eight weeks will be prima facie evidence that the fetus has this capacity, it neither insists that one of that age or more is necessarily viable nor that one which is less mature is, prima facie, non-viable. Viability is a function not only of the fetus itself but also of its environment. A thirty-week fetus born under a hedgerow may well not survive while a proportion of those of twenty-two weeks' gestation would be expected to do so given the availability of a neonatal intensive care unit. Attaining viability thus represents a moment in time which is variable and indeterminable; it follows that it is useless as a measure of the beginning of human life. The term has assumed an irrational importance in the field of fetal rights particularly in the light of the influential US case in 1973 of *Roe* v *Wade*[3]—but note that, even there, the court refused to define 'viability', holding that a matter to be decided by the medical profession. The *fact* of viability, however, has major significance in the management of and legal interpretation of abortion and will be reverted to later in the chapter.

Quickening—that is, the time at which the mother appreciates fetal movement—is, again, so variable and subjective a moment as to be scarcely worth mentioning were it not for its historical interest. For a considerable time, and included in the statute law of England and Wales before 1861,[4] to abort a woman 'quick with child' carried a different penalty from doing so earlier in pregnancy. The concept of quickening as evidence of life does carry the parallel idea of vivification and has some illustrative merit. It is also closely allied to the theories of animation of Aristotle, or of ensoulment as taught by the religious philosophers of the Middle Ages—but these are of more relevance to the later discussion of extra-uterine fertilisation. It is nevertheless clear that quickening is not a moment but part of a process and is correspondingly useless as a marker of human life. Similar criticisms apply to the test of human appearance, which is at the heart of orthodox Jewish teaching. This, however, has greater illustrative significance, particularly from the negative aspect—it is difficult to believe that anyone looking at a twelve-week fetus could *not* appreciate that it was of human form.

The tests of humanity based on segmentation and on the formation of nervous tissue are, again, of greater relevance to the morality of *in vitro* fertilisation and we are left with the widely held and relatively useful criteria of implantation and conception times on which to base an opinion. To regard conception as the point of life at which genetic *homo sapiens* becomes subject to the legal and moral protection afforded to a human being has the attraction of simplicity and the proposition has significant secular support. [5] Belief in conception as the beginning of life is generally attributed to the Roman Catholic church. Even so, the Roman Catholics adopted the proposition only comparatively recently. It was not until 1869 that Pope Pius IX rejected earlier teaching on ensoulment and declared human life to be sacrosanct from the time of conception. [6] It is widely assumed that this change of direction rested on twin pillars—that the development of the infant from a fertilised zygote was demonstrated at that time and that, since the status of a human being was conferred on the fetus at *some* time, it was safer to assume that any fetal rights applied equally to that zygote. The argument is, essentially, taking the continuum theory to its furthest limits: that life is a steady progression from embryo to cadaver. Wennberg[7] points out the logical fallacy behind dependence on such reasoning. By such means, it is as possible to hold that there is no difference between night and day as to believe that embryonic and adult life are of the same quality. The proposition can also be questioned on purely practical grounds. Huge numbers of human zygotes are lost naturally every minute of the day; it seems irrational to attribute humanity to the one which is discovered later and, at the same time, to ignore with equanimity the millions which die unnoticed and unmourned.

The successful zygote, however, is recognisable once it has implanted. At that point, it has a reasonable hold on life; moreover, it is no longer 'external' to its mother[8]—it has become part of the human race both anatomically and physiologically and I shall argue later that it has also acquired a spiritual association. There will be objections that implantation is, itself, a process rather than a sudden change of status. Nevertheless, the successful completion of implantation, even though it is temporary, seems to me to be that point in development at which there is least objection to the attribution of accquired humanity and this is the position which I adopt within the abortion debate.

There are, perhaps, three inevitable sequelae to this conclusion. Firstly, the word humanity is used intentionally. The implanted embryo cannot be seen as a human being. Yet it has acquired humanity and, with that, human rights. Such rights may, in certain circumstances, be subject to those of extant human beings but the closer that embryo comes to the status of a human being—that is, live birth—the less valid is any differential assessment. It follows from this, secondly, that abortion—including displantation—and contraception, are entirely separate and can be distinguished on humanitarian grounds. Abortion destroys humanity and this must be accepted as an absolute in any justification of the procedure. Contraception, although preventing human life, has no destructive element. It is disturbing to find doctors willing to accept such simplistic propositions as: 'essentially any method of contraception is a matter of not wanting the fetus, so it comes down to the question of whether we want contraception. 'Social' abortions are advanced contraception'.[9] Finally, and of major importance, the medical profession is devoted to the service of humanity. Once it is accepted that implantation confers humanity, the abortion debate can be settled by appeal to the Hippocratic conscience. Religious views may have a powerful influence but they are not essential in the medical context.

Legality, practice and morality, are, however, seldom in perfect harmony. We must, therefore, look at these aspects of abortion independently.

Abortion and the law

Contrary to what many doctors would suppose, the law on abortion in England and Wales remains within the Offences Against the Person Act 1861, ss. 58 and 59[10] (Appendix A). The bare bones of the Act are that it is an offence to procure the miscarriage of a woman, to attempt to do so or to supply the means for doing so; the woman herself can only be guilty if she is actually pregnant. Note that the word 'abortion' only appears in the marginal note to the Act; the offence is that of procuring a miscarriage. The law, thus, leaves room for some confusion as to the definition of abortion. Williams[11] defines it as 'feticide: the intentional destruction of the fetus in the womb, or any untimely delivery brought about with intent to cause the death of the fetus' but the Act, as such, carries no indication that this is an essential element. A distinction has been made by the Infant Life (Preservation) Act 1929, which, firstly, introduced the offence of child destruction—that is, killing an infant capable of being born alive; secondly, established the legal presumption that a fetus of twenty-eight weeks' gestation or more is capable of being born alive; and, thirdly, allowed for a defence to child destruction—that the operation was performed in good faith for the purpose of preserving the life of the mother; the defence also exists in Northern Ireland by virtue of the Criminal Justice Act (NI) 1945, s. 25. Apart from the last condition, a legal termination of pregnancy between twenty-eight weeks' gestation and full term must be in the form of an induction of premature labour which is to be distinguished, both medically and legally, from procurement of a miscarriage. Since a fetus of less than twenty-eight weeks' age is progressively less likely to be viable with decreasing maturity, feticide is usually a concomitant of abortion but it is not a primary objective. Advancing medical technology is, however, eroding the limits of fetal viability; fresh problems related to feticide are arising independently of the Abortion Act and will be discussed later, particularly in relation to the living abortus.

It will be seen, therefore, that the Offences Against the Person Act 1861, while being very restrictive as to termination of pregnancy, does not directly address the issues of the quality or the nature of fetal life. It certainly does not equate feticide resulting from abortion with murder, but is simply silent on the subject. The Infant Life (Preservation) Act 1929 is slightly more illuminating in that it specifically values the life of the fetus which is capable of being born alive as being less than that of its mother, given that a choice has to be made. Yet, maintaining its protective purpose it still places a high value on later fetal life. The critical point in the legal devaluation of early fetal life is to be found in the seminal case in 1938 of *R* v *Bourne*[12]—a case which was to have a profound influence within the Commonwealth and throughout the English-speaking world.[13] Mr Bourne, a surgeon of impeccable professional principles, informed the authorities that he intended performing an abortion for a 15-year-old victim of rape and, having done so, was charged under Section 58 of the Offences Against the Person Act 1861. The trial judge, however, applied the enabling provisions of the 1929 Act to the uncompromising 1861 statute. Moreover, he specifically extended the usual interpretation of 'preserving the life of the mother' in saying:

I do not think that it is contended that these words [for the preservation of the life of the mother] mean merely for the preservation of the life of the mother from instant death . . .

and, again:

These words ought to be construed in a reasonable sense and, if the doctor is of the opinion . . . that the probable consequence of the continuance of the pregnancy would be to make the woman a physical or mental wreck, the jury are quite entitled to hold that the doctor who . . . operates is operating for the purpose of preserving the life of the woman.[14]

Mr Bourne was acquitted and this direction remained effectively the English law[15] under which large numbers of therapeutic abortions were performed publicly and without fear of prosecution.[16] A jury decision, however, represents an unsatisfactory flag under which to skirt the criminal law. The reaction of the General Medical Council might also have been unpredictable and there is no doubt that relatively few therapeutic abortions were performed by registered medical practitioners outside specialised units during and shortly after the Second World War. Unplanned pregnancies were probably at their maximum during this period and, consequently, the illegal abortionist thrived. An assessment of the exact extent of the practice is a matter of guess work.[17] There is no doubt that it was widespread but it is interesting that the maximum annual number of deaths due to abortion recorded by the Registrar General for England and Wales before 1968 was 185.

The passage of the Abortion Act 1967 was not only a milestone in British medico-legal history but one which set a precedent throughout the world. The terms of the Act are now so well known as scarcely to merit repetition (it is reproduced in full in Appendix D); the following points are, however, selected for general discussion:

(a) the Act does no more than lay down criteria which elide an offence under the Offences Against the Person Act 1861 when they are observed. It is *not* the definitive law on abortion in Great Britain.[18]

(b) despite appearances to the contrary, the decision to abort is a medical one—taken in good faith by two doctors—rather than that of the woman, whose legal right is to give or withhold consent. The medical profession may be acquiescent but, in theory, the British Act pays no attention to what is termed in the United States 'a woman's constitutional right to privacy'. It has, indeed, been said that the Abortion Act 1967 would be ruled unconstitutional were the three national components of Great Britain to be part of the United States of America.[19]

(c) nevertheless, valid consent to abortion is vested entirely in the mother. The father[20]—who is responsible for fifty per cent of the fetus' genetic constitution—has no legally acceptable contribution to make to the decision.

(d) three of the four main headings under which legal abortion may be performed—the life saving, the health preservation and the social clauses—are orientated towards the well being of the mother; the eugenic clause supposedly concerns the interest of the fetus. Yet the law makes no distinction as to consent to abortion. For reasons which are difficult to understand, the right to die, which is so readily accorded the neonate, is denied to the fetus.[21] The logical conclusion is that the 'eugenic' clause is not there to protect the neonate from a life of pain or mental suffering but rather to insure a mother against the traumas of rearing such an infant—a point which was made many years ago by Havard.[22]

One senses a deep-seated distrust of abortion in the British judiciary. Thus, we have Slade LJ saying that there is nothing in British law to compel a woman to have an abortion.[23] This is unarguably so but, in so saying, he overturned the trial judge's interpretation of a refusal as eliding negligence in a case of failed sterilisation. More definitively Stephenson LJ said:

> To impose such a duty [a right to death] towards the child would be to make a further inroad—in addition to that created by the Abortion Act 1967—into the sanctity of human life which would be contrary to public policy . . .[24]

from which it can certainly be implied that British courts regard fetal life as human life—which they are innately concerned to protect at all levels. The medical profession is, however, motivated by considerations of the overall ill-effects of unwanted pregnancy. It is suspected that doctors in the United States are more polarised in their attitudes to abortion than is the case in Britain and that the process of decriminalisation of abortion in America has derived, in the main, from the efforts of constitutional lawyers rather than from those of the medical profession.

Prior to 1973, the various States of the USA had their own laws which ranged from almost total prohibition of abortion to variations on the English Infant Life (Preservation) Act 1929, the common feature of which was to preserve some intra-uterine fetal rights even when these clashed with those of the mother. Two decisions of the Supreme Court[25] then rendered these unconstitutional. Abortion law in the United States now rests on *Roe* v *Wade* as recently confirmed.[26] The essence of the Supreme Court decision is that it is an invasion of a woman's constitutional right to privacy to limit her access to abortion by statute and there seems no doubt that the result of *Roe* is that termination of pregnancy is a right of the American woman during the first trimester of pregnancy. The State may intervene during the second trimester because it has an interest in the health of the mother; any such action at this point in time is constitutional insofar as it reinforces maternal rights. It is only in the final three months of pregnancy that any fetal rights become recognisable. The State has a compelling interest in the health of the fetus once it is viable—a status which, although regarding it as a purely medical condition, the court assessed as being achieved somewhere between the twenty-fourth and twenty-eighth week of pregnancy. The conceptual difference between the market-forces economy of health care in the United States and the public rights basis of the British National Health Service can, however, be seen in a later Supreme Court decision[27] which limited abortion performed under 'Medicaid' and similar publicly funded schemes to circumstances such as saving the life of the mother or eliminating the effects of rape or incest.

The effect on standards of a combined legal and medical thrust in favour of liberalisation of abortion laws is well seen in Australia where the courts have largely depended upon, and extended, the principles in *Bourne*.[28] Arguing from the premise that anything which is not unlawful (as for example implied in the English Offences Against the Person Act 1861) is likely to be lawful, the jurisdictions of New South Wales and Victoria have established a very liberal approach to abortion.[29] Even so, the effects of the unamended law can still be seen. The doctor performing a therapeutic abortion in Western Australia, for example, still faces the possibility of criminal prosecution. Moreover, court decisions worldwide tend to concentrate on maternal welfare; the legality of abortion for fetal reasons is still doubtful in Australia, except in South Australia and the Northern Territories, in both of which—uniquely—legal abortion is regulated by statute.[30]

Abortion in practice

It is commonly supposed that the demand for abortion is falling off but this is not so. The number of abortions performed in England and Wales in 1986 reached the highest level ever, both in absolute terms—

nearly 172 000 all told—and in rates for resident women in the fertile age group—13.42 per thousand. The most consistently significant age group lies between sixteen to nineteen years, closely run by twenty to twenty-four years: the combined rate for abortion in the two groups in 1986 was approximately twenty-two per thousand women. The comparable figure in the United States is in the region of 1.5 million abortions per annum.

It is certain that the majority of abortion decisions involve the individual woman in an awesome choice. Nevertheless, taken as a whole, the figures suggest an acceptance on the part of the general public of the taking of fetal life which occurs on the scale of deaths arising from a major wartime operation. The medical profession has, in general, tended to see any shortcomings in the Abortion Act in terms of inadequate facilities in the National Health Service;[31] and the run of the mill general practitioner is now quoted: 'If abortion is available, I think that giving the choice to the mother is for the increasing good of society and for the benefit of children . . . Abortion is part of the spectrum of our society, enhancing society'.[32]

It is difficult to believe that the original drafters of the Abortion Act 1967 envisaged the operation being undertaken on such a scale and doubts must be raised as to whether the condition of medical 'good faith' inserted in s. 1(1) of the Act is being disregarded. If it is, it would be most likely to show up in abortions performed outwith the National Health Service for health reasons—which include psychological health—and especially in those performed on non-resident women. In 1986, fifty per cent of abortions on resident women were performed under the aegis of the National Health Service; the figure for non-residents was 0.32 per cent. In the same year, eighty-eight per cent of abortions on resident women were for health reasons as compared with ninety-seven per cent in non-residents. In contrast, abortions performed for fetal reasons—which can be taken to be the ground for which there is most scientifically proven justification—comprised 1.3 per cent of NHS abortions, 0.35 per cent of private 'resident' examinations and 0.17 per cent of all non-resident cases.

The figures speak for themselves yet there appears to be only one case reported in the United Kingdom of a doctor being prosecuted under the Abortion Act 1967 and this was on the grounds of how, rather than why, the operation was performed.[33] The same benign attitude to the medical profession is shown in countries where legal abortion is not defined by statute as is the case in most States of Australia, where there have been no prosecutions of doctors since 1971. The reasons for this general immunity are complex but must, to a large extent, depend upon the near impossibility of defining or of proving *bad* faith, and on the ever widening interpretation of what is 'not unlawful'. Thus, in the English case of *R v Newton and Stungo*, 1958,[34] the already stretched definition of preserving the life of the mother was further extended to mean no more than preserving physical or mental health; this pattern has been followed judicially in Victoria and New South Wales.[35] The onus which rests on the prosecution to prove beyond reasonable doubt that an abortion was performed in the absence of honest belief in its therapeutic value is now so great that criminal trials would be pointless.

There is, however, a hint of a groundswell towards greater acknowledgement of fetal rights, particularly in the later stages of pregnancy. This manifests itself through calls for the amendment of the Infant Life (Preservation) Act 1929, to lower the gestational age at which there is a presumption of capacity to be born alive. A further Infant Life (Preservation) Bill was introduced in the House of Lords in 1987; the Select Committee of the House of Lords has now recommended that the Bill should not proceed but that the Abortion Act 1967, s.1 should be amended so that, after 24 weeks' gestation, termination should not be permitted unless two registered medical practitioners are of the opinion that the termination is essential to the woman's physical or mental health and that late abortions should not be performed on the ground only of risk to the physical or mental health of any existing members of the family.[36] Parallel with this, the Abortion (Amendment) Bill 1987 —which seeks to limit to 18 weeks the gestational age at which legal terminations can be performed other than for the purpose of saving the life of or preventing grave permanent injury to the health of the woman —is before the House of Commons; despite considerable support for the measure, it is unlikely that it will be enacted without significant alteration. One counter to such proposals is that the intra-uterine diagnosis of congenital defect is time consuming; a reduction in the age limit for legal abortion would, therefore, jeopardise that ground for legal abortion which many would regard as being readily acceptable. The figures show that there is some basis for this concern. The proportion of all abortions performed for fetal reasons on residents of England and Wales in 1986 was 1.3 per cent. If, however, abortions beyond the twentieth week of pregnancy are considered alone, the proportion is eighteen per cent—a figure which has been rising, presumably due to the greater variety and complexity of investigations becoming available. The significance of this massive discrepancy will be reverted to in chapter 9; for the present, it is only suggested that the statistics indicate that there are conceptual, legal and practical reasons for separating fetal from maternal grounds for abortion.

The morality of abortion

Once the concept that humanity begins with implantation is admitted, the need for an acceptable moral justification for abortion increases. A major apologist for the practice is Glover who considers all requested abortions to be morally justified on the grounds that there should be as few unwanted children as possible.[37] The main general argument to be used *against* abortion, says Glover, is that it reduces the number of worthwhile persons; he has also pointed out that fetuses are, in the main, easily replaceable. On this basis, contraception and abortion are equally moral.

This argument has an elegant simplicity and a somewhat rugged practicality. But, as Glover explains, it depends on confining one's analysis to the 'direct' effects of abortion. In practice, different 'side' effects will stem from the two approaches to planned parenthood. In this respect he lists the side effects of abortion on the mother herself, on the medical staff and on society at large. Contraception and abortion cannot be equated when these are taken into consideration; moreover, a qualitative difference between early and late abortions is exposed—the later the abortion, the worse are the side effects.

Looked at in this light, all abortions of unwanted fetuses are morally justified in themselves; fetal development is a continuum which is of significance only insofar as it affects others. No attention is paid to the fetus whose increasing rights, if any, are ill-defined. Opposing suggestions such as that which holds that human life depends upon 'brain possession' have the alternative merit that they simultaneously define a fetus which is without 'life' and one which has the attributes of humanity.[38] The door is thus opened to distinguishing abortions to which there can be no moral objection from those which involve the taking of human life. I, on the other hand, have argued that the crucial point in fetal development lies at implantation and acceptance of this carries the implication that *any* abortion must involve the destruction of human life. Each operation has to be justified with this factor in one of the balance pans, for the morality of an abortion depends upon how the balance lies between the rights of one who has an unexpressed humanity and those of one who has the undeniable advantage of the obvious status of a human being. Each merits some discussion.

Maternal rights

Demands to change the abortion laws are grounded in the claim that it is a woman's right to choose. This contention is associated, in its most extreme form of expression, with the concept of self-defence—the mother is entitled to defend herself against an intruder who threatens her.

Self-defence is clearly a reason for abortion in any case where the mother's life is clearly threatened. The principle becomes less acceptable, however, when it is extended to include threats to an undefinable state of health. Once such extrapolation is admitted, the road is open to trade fetal life against lesser factors such as maternal psychological inconvenience. There is evidence that this occurs in practice, Peel, for example, being quoted as saying that most abortions are totally unrelated to physical or mental health.[39] There is, moreover, something distasteful in the suggestion of conflict between mother and fetus and one wonders if it might not, in fact, be being over-played. Medical experience is that most mothers will fight to retain babies who are clearly threatening them through, say, toxaemia of pregnancy. It is likely that the majority of the relatively few abortions performed in order to preserve the life of the mother (480 in women residents in England and Wales in 1986) were undertaken contrary to the mothers' preferences; certainly there were 147619 legal abortions on residents of England and Wales in 1986 but, at the same time, there were 661018 live births. McLean and Maher[40] point out that 'it is the evil intent on the part of the assailant which explains the moral permissibility of self defence'; if intent is to be attributed to the fetus, it must also be allowed autonomy—and that would make self-defence a self-defeating argument for those who wish to exclude the fetus from decision-making as to its fate.

A less combative justification of the right to choose lies in the principle of maternal autonomy—the right to dispose of her body as she selects—or, in transatlantic terms, on the right to personal privacy. This is sometimes expressed in somewhat shrill terms:

The increasing tendency to view the fetus as an independent patient or person occurs at the cost of reducing the woman to the status of little more than a maternal environment . . . The need is to reform the right to abortion as one not to be defined by the fetus or by technological advances but one that is tied to women's constitutional rights to privacy, autonomy and bodily integrity.[41]

A more disarming approach is that of Thomson[42] who maintains that the mother's right to control her own body overrides the right to life of the fetus unless the mother has a special responsibility to it. Such a responsibility would exist if the parents had in no way tried to prevent its existence; but when they have taken reasonable contraceptive precautions, they cannot be said to have assumed responsibility for an unwelcome consequence and, in these circumstances, the fetus has no right to the use of the mother's body.

This view presupposes that the decision over parenthood has been taken after due consideration. Useful though it is, the proposition does nothing to assist in the case of those who have been reckless as to the result of sexual intercourse. To refuse abortion in these circumstances would be punitive and the suggestion falls short of its primary purpose for that reason. It does, however, provide a clear justification for termination of a pregnancy following rape, incest or, since a minor under 16 is legally incapable of consent to sexual intercourse, of any pregnancy in a girl below the age of sixteen—categories which, unusually, are not specifically delineated in United Kingdom legislation.

It is just possible to extend such categories of 'unwanted' babies to include those of uncaring parents. But to do so would be to regard abortion and contraception as comparable—which may be an arguable view but one which is unacceptable to me. The fetus must be thought of as more than a mere appendage to its mother; to argue the contrary is to ignore an individual's genetic constitution, for the mother and her fetus *are* genetically distinct. It would be unrealistic to deny some sympathy for the extreme view that the fetus is a parasite but, in allowing this, it must also be accepted that it is not a self-aggressive parasite—its situation results from an invitation issued, maybe grudgingly or even unwillingly, by the mother. The woman's choice whether or not to invite *conception* can be made independently of any other existing interests. After implantation, the rights of a second party who has, at least, a potential for autonomy, have also to be considered. And, to quote again from McLean and Maher,[43] no disrespect is shown for the mother by then denying abortion unless it can be shown that she should not be held responsible for being pregnant. The issue that the so-called 'pro-choice' position fails to meet is whether a woman, in exercising what she regards as a right to expel an unwanted fetus, also has a *right* to, as opposed to a necessary acceptance of, the death of that fetus. The problem will be looked at later in relation to the living abortus.

Fetal rights

Although I have tried to establish that, following implantation, the fetus has humanity, this is not to say it has the full autonomy of a human being—it would be almost indefensible to hold that it has. On the other hand, it clearly has potential autonomy and its rights vis à vis the autonomy of its mother depend upon the strength of that potential.

Theoretically, this potential for autonomy is identical in the zygote and in the full term fetus which it is to become. But to hold that this conclusion must be followed in practice is to deny the obvious—that, given the option of abortion, the weight given to the humanity of the fetus in decision making must increase with its physical development. This apparent contradiction can be explained by consideration of how likely it is that the potential for autonomy will mature. Thus, there is very little certainty that the newly implanted embryo will achieve the full autonomy of a separate existence but, once viability is reached, the potential to do so is unmistakable. It may, indeed, be as obvious as that, having reached the third trimester, the fetus can rightly be regarded as having an autonomy equal to that of its mother.

In the United Kingdom, the evidence in favour of this view is somewhat static and negative insofar as the Infant Life (Preservation) Act 1929 does no more than limit the grounds for a legal abortion after the twenty-eighth week of pregnancy to saving the life of the mother. The trend towards accepting the gestational development of some fetal autonomy is more positive and dynamic in the United States. Thus, even in the sensational case of *Roe* v *Wade*,[44] it was held that the State had a compelling interest to intervene in an abortion issue on behalf of the fetus once it had reached viability—subject only to the condition of saving the life of the mother. In 1981,[45] the Supreme Court of Georgia went so far as to order a caesarian section to protect the life of the viable fetus of a woman who refused operation on religious grounds. The legality of this decision was not tested because the mother's condition righted itself spontaneously. In *Taft* v *Taft*,[46] the trial court ruled that a husband had authority to consent to treatment on behalf of his wife in order to insure against likely miscarriage. Admittedly, the Massachusetts Supreme Court reversed this decision but, in doing so, it left open the possibility of ordering a pregnant woman to submit to a surgical procedure in order to protect a *viable* fetus. The court also distinguished between surgical and medical treatment and reserved judgment on whether there might be justification for ordering the latter to protect the non-viable fetus: 'the State's interest in some circumstances might be sufficiently compelling to justify restriction of a person's constitutional right of privacy'.[46]

There is indirect evidence for an increasing acceptance of fetal rights in the United Kingdom, Canada and, possibly, the United States[47] which derives from the concept of child abuse during pregnancy through drug taking;[48] but, undoubtedly, the most important catalyst in this reaction is the growing realisation that the fetus may take on the status of a patient in its own right. Keyserlingk, in particular, has stressed the need for the same legal protections and interventions for fetuses as are attributable to children, his argument resting particularly on the grounds that there is a continuance between the two states.[49]

It is, however, widely held that the severely defective fetus loses potential autonomy in direct relationship to its degree of disability and, from that, it is extrapolated that the mother has an equivalent linear right to abortion when carrying a defective child.[50] This view which, as has been discussed, is inherent in the maternally orientated Abortion Act, has been accepted by religious leaders[51] and, at least by implication, by the law.[52] I would suggest, however, that it is better, on both moral and practical grounds, to agree with Ramsey[53] and to isolate abortion on the grounds of fetal abnormality in a separate category of fetal euthanasia. Termination of pregnancy on fetal grounds should be regarded as a surrogate expression of a fetal right—one to be exercised in the best interests of a fetus just as it should be exercised on behalf of the neonate in the practice of selective non-treatment of the newborn. The matter is specifically discussed in chapter 9.

The outcome of all the variables discussed must lie in the compromise proposition that, while the mother has no inherent moral right to an abortion, there is, at the same time, no absolute right to fetal survival in a hostile maternal environment. Abortion on demand is unacceptable once humanity is accorded the implanted fetus but, in the event of maternal/fetal conflict, fetal rights increase with fetal development so that feticide is justifiable only in exceptional circumstances after the attainment of what, for want of a better term, we may call viability. At the other extreme, it may be that there is no moral turpitude in the destruction of an unimplanted embryo. Yet, here, the drafting of the Abortion Act is such that this apparently innocuous action may be illegal. A consideration of abortion and its impact on the sanctity of life doctrine would be incomplete without some discussion of these two diametrically opposed conditions.

The living abortus

As discussed, the limits of viability are being pushed back in the gestational scale. This is not due to any physiological changes in the fetus but rather to the continuing advances of paediatric intensive care. Many premature infants are born alive but whether they are 'viable' depends on the availability of modern technology and on the willingness of doctors to use extreme measures in the individual case.

Approximately 4.8 per cent of abortions are carried out in England and Wales when the fetus is of nineteen weeks' gestation or older—a total of 8365 in 1986. Certainly, a proportion of these are 'capable of being born alive'—that is, capable of breathing either with or without ventilator support—and these are theoretically protected by the Infant Life (Preservation) Act 1929. The statute makes no distinction as to whether the abortus dies *in utero* or following extraction. There is, on the other hand, a marked practical difference. While it may never be known if the child which died *in utero* was capable of being born alive, there can be no doubt when death occurs on the sluice-room table, and it is at this point that the door to a charge of homicide is opened. An abortus born alive has the same legal rights as does any premature infant[54] and it follows that successful action taken to kill such a subject potentially qualifies as either murder or manslaughter. On the other hand, should the fetus live despite an intention that it should die during the process of abortion, there is the chance, admittedly improbable, of a charge of attempted child destruction.[55]

The major difficulty facing the obstetrician is that, while he is performing a legal termination under the Abortion Act 1967, he cannot, because of its loose wording, be certain whether or not he is committing an offence under the 1929 Act until the abortion is complete. The important case of C v S has at least clarified that a live birth must include a physiological ability to breathe. The argument as to the relevance of the 1929 Act (protecting a fetus 'capable of being born alive') and the 1967 Act ('preserving the life of a viable foetus') is now largely settled.[56]

There is a great deal to be said for a comprehensive review of, and integration of, the Offences Against the Person Act 1861, the Infant Life (Preservation) Act 1929 and the Abortion Act 1967 but, currently, the obstetrician must take his chance with the law as it stands and, as it stands, he is likely to choose methods of abortion which ensure a dead abortus. Feticide is thus sought not, primarily, for the benefit of the mother nor for the interests of the fetus but, rather, for the protection of the doctor. Sometimes, indeed, this may result in disadvantage to the mother, as when intra-amniotic saline infusions are chosen in preference to the less toxic prostaglandins; in addition, conditions which ensure death of the fetus may be offensive to the nursing staff, as when dilatation and evacuation, which involves severe fetal trauma, is chosen. The issue has been expressly met in the United States where a statute, requiring persons performing abortions to adhere to a prescribed standard of care if the fetus is or may be viable, has been declared unconstitutional. The possibility of criminal proceedings was thought likely to have a chilling effect on the willingness of physicians to perform abortions near viability and would, thus, encroach upon women's rights. [57]

Opposing views may, however, prevail in countries other than the United States. The Lane Committee (reporting, admittedly, as long ago as 1974) stated:

> It is unlawful for termination of pregnancy to be carried out by a method which destroys a fetus capable of being born alive, even if its chances of survival are slight or non-existent . . . If an alive and apparently viable fetus emerges from the termination there is a statutory duty to try and keep it alive . . . Further, if after delivery a fetus shows signs of life, an offence is committed if its birth and death are not registered or if it is incinerated other than in a crematorium. [58]

Somerville, writing from Canada, [59] believed that the physician not only had no right to kill a fetus unnecessarily but that he is legally obligated not to do so. Morally, I must agree with this. It may be that the preservation of life is no longer the major function of the medical profession, but the only objective which would take precedence would be the relief of suffering. There is no mandate to allow a 'person in being' to die who is either not suffering or whose suffering could be assuaged by an oxygen-rich environment. There can be few processes more contrary to the Hippocratic principle, nor to which the word 'brutalisation' can be better applied, than that of allowing a newly born infant to die in the sink. Yet what is the doctor to do faced with such a situation? He has, effectively, contracted with the mother to relieve her of her infant; he cannot simply hand it back to her with apologies nor can he assure the infant of a loving adoptive environment should he or she survive.

Therein lies a further dilemma. As already noted, some eighteen per cent of late abortions are performed for fetal reasons and both the proportion and the numbers are likely to rise with increasing availability of diagnostic techniques. Thus, the obstetrician faced with a living abortus may not only be required to make a life or death decision but also to base that decision on an assessment of the quality of that life—an assessment which must be made, this time, without parental help. And, as if the catalogue of quandaries was not already long enough, prematurity carries hazards of its own irrespective of apparent normality or abnormality at birth. Thus, nineteen per cent of long term survivors following birth between the gestational ages of twenty-three to twenty-eight weeks were found to have physical impairments which, presumably, resulted from that prematurity.[60]

There is little wonder that the law treads warily in this clinical and ethical minefield. There have been a number of unsuccessful prosecutions in the United States, the best known on this side of the Atlantic being that of Dr Waddill. Waddill ordered 'oxygen-only' for a 26-week-old fetus who survived a saline-infusion abortion. On its death, he was charged with murder and the trial ended with a jury divided 7:5 in favour of acquittal. A second trial to which he was subjected also resulted in a 'hung jury', at which point the judge dismissed all criminal charges against him.[61] Most instances which have come to notice in the United Kingdom have done so through the medium of the Coroner's court and are, consequently, poorly reported and are of no precedental value. To the best of my knowledge, only one coroner has attributed death in such circumstances to want of attention at the birth of a premature infant[62] and there was no subsequent legal action. Dr Hamilton, who was accused of having abandoned an abortus which turned out, unexpectedly, to be of thirty weeks' gestation, was charged with attempted murder at the instigation of the Director of Public Prosecutions. The Magistrates' Court took the unusual step of declaring that there was no case to answer and, accordingly, the matter did not go before a jury.[63]

Yet one feels that the law has got to face this issue at some time. Better than leaving it to be decided in courts, this would be a suitable area to include in an overall legislative review of the status of the embryo, the fetus and the neonate, as was suggested by the Warnock Committee (see chapter 8). Some personal views on possible legislation are offered in chapter 9.

The unimplanted embryo

There has been considerable academic discussion as to whether the use of methods calculated to prevent implantation of the fertilised ovum—for example, the use of certain post-coital hormones or the fitting of an intra-uterine device—constitute procuring a miscarriage. The debate has been given greater emphasis because of its relation to *in vitro* fertilisation, but I regard it as being, to an extent, unnecessarily prolonged. From the moral point of view, it is clear that, since I do not regard humanity as being acquired until implantation is achieved, I do not see the extraction of an unimplanted embryo as involving human life. Secondly, even if it is held that humanity begins with conception, interception of the unimplanted embryo must be that method of terminating pregnancy which, by any standards, is the least distasteful. Thirdly, there is the near impossibility of proving the fact of interception in the individual case—so much so that the methods could not possibly be unlawful in Scotland.[64] And, from the legal point of view, the Attorney General is quoted as saying that:

The phrase procure a miscarriage cannot be construed to include the prevention of implantation . . . The ordinary use of the word miscarriage [in the nineteenth century] referred to interference at a later stage of pre-natal development than implantation.[65]

While this does not carry judicial weight, it is very persuasive.

These comments were made in response to referrals of cases to the Law Officers and it is therefore still possible that the issue may reassume practical significance. It is reasonable to hold that, if the Attorney General is wrong, both the woman who accepts and the doctor who prescribes interceptive methods of preventing pregnancy could be guilty, respectively, of contravening s.58 and s.59 of the Offences Against the Person Act 1861. The matter turns on two questions—first, whether abortion and miscarriage are synonomous and, second, if so, whether one can procure the miscarriage of a woman whose fetus is not yet implanted.

There are good reasons for distinguishing abortion and miscarriage medically but a case can be made for regarding the terms as being interchangeable in law.[66] Indeed, despite the semantic difficulties resulting from later legislation, they were so used in the Act of 1803.[67] The answer to the question, however, is by no means fully agreed.[68] One way of resolving the matter may be through considering the second question. To argue that a woman is 'carrying' an unimplanted fetus is to ignore the point already made that structures or substances present within those body cavities which have openings to the outside are anatomically 'external' to the body. There can be no true carriage of something which has a high probability of slipping away and it follows that there can be no miscarriage until the embryonic tissue is integrated with that of the mother either by implantation or through the placenta. The pre-implantation embryo may be waiting for the bus but it is not yet being carried on its platform.

It is almost inconceivable that the law would risk ridicule by prosecuting a woman who wears an IUD or takes a 'morning-after pill'. The doctor, however, is in a more vulnerable position because the essence of an offence in his case lies in intent. There is no need to prove, either physiologically or semantically, that the woman was 'with child' when he intended to abort that child before a prosecution can succeed under s.59 of the 1861 Act. Moreover, as things stand, he commits an offence under the 1967 Act if he is uncertain of the fact of pregnancy. Accordingly, the Lane Committee[69] recommended that the statute be amended so as to read additionally: 'reference to termination of pregnancy

includes acts done with intent to terminate a pregnancy if such exists'.
On the medical side, it has been recommended that, to be safe from the
law, interceptive methods should not be undertaken more than seventy-
two hours after sexual intercourse.[68]

The reason for this is, of course, that conditions change dramatically
once implantation has occurred (usually thought to be around the eighth
day). Interceptive methods then become displanting methods and it is
unarguable that an abortion is either being attempted or performed in
such circumstances—there is no logical reason why a similar operation
with similar objectives should change its legal nature because it is
performed at two rather than twelve weeks' gestation. Thus, although it
may be the least emotionally unacceptable form of abortion, it would
seem that the quaintly named 'menstrual extraction' is certainly unlawful unless performed in accordance with the Abortion Act 1967, s.1[70]
and it may be so even then, without a change in the wording of the
statute. The whole subject is, however, one which is better considered as
an aspect of embryocide.

8. Embryocide

In considering the values which are placed on human lives, we have worked backwards from those who are close to death to those existing as an early fetus. Until a few years ago this would have sufficed to cover the span of human life. Now, faced with the rapid development of new reproductive technologies, consideration has to be given to the existence of, and consequent moral implications of, extra-uterine or *in vitro* embryos which have a human genetic constitution. It is important to appreciate that any problems which arise do so not from improper motives but from the laudable objectives of research into genetic disease and of treating those forms of infertility which are caused by abnormalities in the female. The need for such treatment is said to occur in some five per cent of marriages in which a family is wanted.

The practical difficulty which creates the moral problem is, perhaps, by now so well understood as scarcely to merit recapitulation. In essence, it rests on the fact that some surplus embryos must be formed in the laboratory if treatment is to be maximally effective. This need arises in a progressive mode: a number of embryos must be introduced into the uterus in order to increase the likelihood of one implantation; a larger number of ova than will be needed must be impregnated *in vitro* so as to allow for failure to produce or for the formation of defective embryos. Since few biological equations are perfect, a successful *in vitro* fertilisation must result in an excess of embryos.

Put simply like this, it does not seem to be a matter of great consequence. An untold number of human spermatozoa and very large numbers of ova are formed and passed without maturing into an adult human being; does it matter if, in the course of this fruitless existence, some of them have fused during the process? The majority of natural conceptuses are lost before they are implanted—should it be a cause for concern that some are formed and die with no attempt having been made to achieve that implantation? The answer is, of course, that these are matters of very great moment to those who believe that humanity, with its attendant rights, begins at conception. Given that belief, an embryo *in vitro* deserves as much respect as does one *in utero* and, therefore, according to the same belief, as much as does an adult human being. But, at the other end of the spectrum, there are those who see no moral value in a microscopic collection of undifferentiated cells whose greatest claim to humanhood would be to give a positive reaction to anti-human antiserum.

The solution to the inevitable clashes of opinion as to the nature of the *in vitro* embryo has exercised the minds of government-established committees on both sides of the Atlantic and throughout the Commonwealth. In the United States, the Ethics Advisory Board[1] was quite open in regarding the moral status of the embryo and the ethics of the consequential potential for research on *in vitro* embryos as being among the most difficult they had confronted. These same difficulties caused great divisions among the members of the British Warnock Committee[2] and, considering the complexities involved, it is surprising how similar were both the approaches and the conclusions of these two influential bodies.

Both saw a need for compromise. In the United States, it was said:

The human embryo is entitled to profound respect but this respect does not necessarily encompass the full legal and moral rights attributable to persons . . .

while the Warnock Committee recommended only that the embryo of the human species should be afforded *some* protection in law (my emphasis). The practical compromise recommendation reached in both Britain and America was that the unimplanted human embryo may be violated up to, but not beyond, fourteen days' development.

There are good anatomical and physiological reasons for regarding this as an appropriate cut-off point. It is at about this time that identifiable embryonic structures appear within the developing cell mass, that twinning becomes no longer possible, that specialised fetal growth begins and that the successful embryo developing *in vivo* (in the living body) would certainly have implanted. Good as these reasons may be, it is clear that the recommendation derived is purely empirical. Embryonic development is a process involving the replication of human genetic material which is of identical structure irrespective of the precise moment of development. There is no reason why human material of thirteen days' age should be protected any more or any less than that which is fifteen days old.[3] Devices which disguise this fact—such as the use of the term 'pre-embryo' to isolate the embryo which has no anatomical differentiation—have been expressly said not to imply any moral evaluation.[4] It becomes, surely, a matter of a clear-cut, yes or no, decision—either the *in vitro* embryo of *Homo sapiens* is a human being with rights that are absolute in themselves, and which only become comparative when they are in conflict with those of human beings in a more developed state, or it is an artefact to be regarded in the same light as any other biological product of the laboratory. There is no place for such musings as: 'human embryo has a value of something more than that of a mouse embryo but rather less than that of a human fetus'.[5] The Warnock Committee does seem to have been at odds with itself on this point; whereas they concluded that the human *in vitro* embryo was entitled to some respect, they recommended, in fact, to confer *full* respect on that which was more than fourteen days old but none, other than the protection of a licence, to that which was younger. It has to be seen whether there are any legal or more certain moral indicators of the *in vitro* embryo's true position.

Legal assistance

At the time of writing, there is no law relating to the *in vitro* embryo comparable to that which surrounds the *in vivo* fetus. Indeed, the Warnock Committees' plea for a comprehensive review of the law relating to all stages of human development prior to birth was that part of its report which, in the opinion of many, attracted greatest sympathy. It seemed to the Committee to be illogical:

> to propose stringent legislative controls on the use of very early human embryos for research, while there is a less formal mechanism governing the research use of whole live embryos and fetuses of more advanced gestation. [6]

No one could fail to agree with this but, meantime, in the absence of specific legislation on the point, indications as to the probable state of the law must be extracted from that which exists.

If we assume that the *in vitro* embryo is a human being in possession of all the rights which that entails, then it follows that its deliberate destruction is murder, and that conclusion is plainly absurd. It is ridiculous to stretch the imagination into regarding the destruction of a microscopic sixteen-cell morula as the killing of a reasonable creature in being. It is, indeed, difficult to see what offence could possibly be committed in so doing. It is clearly not an offence against the Offences Against the Person Act 1861, s.58 because that entails the procuring, or the attempted procuring, of a miscarriage of a woman. There is, at the moment, no offence of embryocide because the concept is novel to the law; similarly, there is no offence of feticide *per se* because, as discussed in the previous chapter, actions against the fetus are related to its mother in both a restrictive and an enabling sense. No way can be envisaged by which current United Kingdom law could justify a prosecution for the destruction of *in vitro* embryos.

The question can also be looked at from the negative aspect. If the law is happy, through increasingly liberal abortion regulations, to adopt an increasingly acquiescent attitude to the destruction of a fetus which has a recognisable hold on life, why should it concern itself with structures which, currently, have no potential for full development unless assisted by the technology of the obstetric laboratory? In practical terms, a dismissive answer would seem appropriate yet, such is the public concern, that there is significant pressure in favour of legislative intervention at this level.

As a result, two bills have been introduced to Parliament which have sought to make it a criminal offence to fertilise an ovum *in vitro* unless it is to be implanted in a uterus. These bills received surprising support and were defeated only on procedural grounds. Many of the United States have either introduced specific legislation or have relied upon existing Child Abuse Acts to protect the *in vitro* embryo. [8] The Australian state of Victoria, which harbours what is, perhaps, the most advanced *in vitro* fertilisation programme in the world, has recently passed restrictive legislation[9] of which it has been said—perhaps erroneously—that it will inhibit the development of therapy for the infertile in favour of the 'rights' of the embryo. [10] The political tears shed on behalf of surplus embryos which are to be counted annually in dozens look suspiciously crocodile when contrasted with the dry eyes which contemplate 170000 legal abortions in Great Britain each year. And, to add a final legal comment, once it is agreed that pre-implantation methods of contraception are lawful, and, as discussed above, it is almost certain that they are at least not unlawful, it would seem that any attempt to define a legal source of protection for the embryo is little more than casuistry.

The moral status of the embryo

The law being unhelpful, one has to turn to moralists for guidance as to the intrinsic value of the embryo—but here, again, there is little unanimity. Those who are attracted to the concept of 'personhood' clearly have no difficulty; if rights and respect depend upon self-expression or self-determination, then there is little which could be less deserving of either than the *in vitro* embryo. At the other end of the scale, however,

> Those who find it ethically acceptable not to take the level of development into account when weighing the claims of an adult woman and her family against those of a not yet conscious fetus will never accept that uniqueness [as a human being] is the only relevant factor. [11]

A belief that humanity and human dignity begin with conception leads to the inevitable conclusion that the only logical answer is to ban all *in vitro* reproductive technology because embryo wastage and the treatment of infertility in the female are inseparable. The apologist for such therapy is, therefore, exposed to a charge of attempted retrospective moral justification of a practice which has already evolved and is being widely practised. [12] To be credible, he must establish a deontological argument for distinguishing the *in vitro* embryo from the human person. To achieve this involves, first, considering the position of the major opposition which is represented most emphatically by orthodox Roman Catholic teaching. [13] This may be summarised by taking a number of quotations from a highly persuasive paper by Iglesias:[14]

> To be a human being is to be a person. There are no stages in our existence at which this identity does not hold . . .
> If we are to make sense of our existence *now* as human personal

beings we must admit that whatever capacities we have now have developed from what we were in the beginning . . .

Respect due to the human embryo must not differ *in kind* from the respect due to any other human being; the human embryo must be protected as a human being, not as a property or an object of use . . .

The fact that the zygote is a living being from conception onwards is a sufficient reason for many to recognise that it must be treated and protected not as property but as a member of the human family.

These are abstract philosophical concepts but, given that there are no practical grounds on which to determine the morality or immorality of embryocide, one has to depend upon such considerations. It is presumptuous and, to say the least, foolhardy to appear to argue religious morals with the Vatican Congregation for the Doctrine of the Faith. Nevertheless, I suggest that there is a counter argument to that explained by Iglesias which starts from the premise that there is nothing *material* within the animal kingdom, other than the precise structure of the relevant genes, which distinguishes the species *Homo sapiens* from, say, *Gorilla gorilla*. The justification of so-called 'speciesism' depends upon some particular quality or qualities of the human being. Iglesias listed these as including self-consciousness, self-determination, responsibility, love and creativity. These properties can be summarised as representing the 'soul' of man which distinguishes his spiritual and cultural isolation from other animals. It is this concept of ensoulment which, as discussed under abortion, was once taken to justify the demarcation of the early from the late fetus and which has, latterly, been transferred to the point of conception. There are reasonable grounds for assuming that at least part of the reason for this movement from the early Aquinian view, which measured the pre-ensoulment phase in terms of weeks, was dictated by advances in medical and scientific knowledge[15] but, as Dunstan has pointed out, dependence on such shifting ground may be a two-edged sword—a firm line must be drawn at some point.

I have already discussed my reasons for believing that humanity begins with implantation of the embryo and I suggest that the same arguments can be extended to cover the spiritual field as well. If humanity and ensoulment are interdependent, in my view it follows that implantation, rather than conception, is also the logical point in human development to which ensoulment can be attributed. From which it follows that the *in vitro* embryo, which has never known a womb, has neither the physical nor the spiritual attributes of humanity but that, once implanted, the *in vivo* embryo derives these from its mother.

Acceptance of this 'theological' theory has an obvious, and important, practical corollary—the ethical doubts surrounding *in vitro* fertilisation are, thereby, eliminated. Destruction of the *in vitro* embryo involves no attack on the sanctity of human life because the *in vitro* embryo has no humanity. Naturally this approach attracts considerable criticism. Its most obvious failure is that its valid application depends on the sophistication of technology and may, therefore, be only temporary; it would, for example, disintegrate were it possible to develop the embryo to the stage of an in vitro full term fetus. One would then be confronted with the contradiction in terms of a soulless human being. Happily, it can be said that such a day is in the far distant future; but, having reached that conclusion, which must seem unsatisfactory to many, it is comforting to find the Jesuit philosopher Rahner accepting that, whereas a different judgment may be shown to be correct at a later time, 'a particular contingent judgment can still be the only correct one in its situation'. [16]

Nonetheless, this criticism serves to emphasise the importance of placing some time limit on the lawful development of the human species in vitro. This is not particularly important for the purposes of the present discussion of the value of 'human' life—the death of an embryo should have the same intrinsic significance irrespective of its age. Rather, it must be accepted that the longer the time available for manipulation and the more developed the embryo which is being 'used', the greater will be the public sense of misgiving as to what is involved in the wider sense. As Lady Warnock has written: 'people generally believe that science may be up to no good, and must not be allowed to proceed without scrutiny, both of its objectives and of its methods'. [17]

This leads to a consideration of the morality of the production and destruction of human embryos purely for the purposes of research and experimentation, a matter which seriously split the Warnock Committee. Ostensibly, there is little difference between using and destroying one embryo which could have been, but was not, selected for therapy of the infertile and another which was produced independently of any treatment schedule. As the majority of the Committee thought (at para 11.28): 'in neither case would (the embryos) have a potential for life because in neither case were they to be transferred to a uterus'. Yet, despite the strong logic of this reasoning, many would see the two processes as lying on different moral planes. I would admit to being in their ranks and, given my analysis of the status of the in vitro embryo, there is a strong possibility that I am being inconsistent in adopting such a position. Where, it will be asked, does the difference lie if neither has humanity?

It is possible to justify this stance on grounds which are more acceptable than those of mere intuition. There are good reasons for doubting the morality of producing any biological material simply in order to destroy it; and, again at the risk of being accused of 'speciesism', it would be unreal not to admit that human biological material has a special position. Its creation must, therefore, be particularly well justified. At present, it is very doubtful if the consequentialist argument—to the effect that the greater good will derive from the use of the research potential within the embryonic structures—is sufficient justification for their deliberate construction and destruction in the cause of experimentation. On the other hand, the provision of a potential treatment for tens of thousands of British women does seem a good end which should be sought if so doing is consonant with both the laws and the morals of society. So long as that is the end in view, it is possible to apply a modified doctrine of 'double effect' (see p. 18).

The production of surplus embryos may be undesirable but is bound to occur within this acceptable therapeutic regime. Since it is not rational to expect receptive wombs to be available for all of them, there is no alternative, in the end, to their destruction. Greater benefit will result if they contribute to the future health of the population through the medium of research before reaching the inevitable conclusion. But no such principle can be applied to the production of embryos which are not intended for treatment; instead, the spectre is raised of the dedicated scientist experimenting for the sake of experimentation within a moral minefield. It is interesting to note that Steptoe, the British pioneer of in vitro fertilisation, did not deliberately create embryos for research,[18] but it has to be appreciated that he was in clinical practice and that this denial of a research potential does not imply that the practice is not being adopted in academic institutions.

Even so, clinical practice raises its own related problems which, although referable to the abortion debate, are best discussed within the framework of the in vitro fertilisation programme. There seems little doubt that the success of in vitro fertilisation is, to an extent, proportional to the number of zygotes that are introduced to the recipient womb. Nature itself regulates the outcome in the great majority of cases but, occasionally, the procedure is so successful that multiple pregnancies occur—sometimes to the extent of sextuplet or septuplet implantations.

The pragmatic response to such an event depends upon the position from which the view is taken. From the economic and social aspect, the 'best' outcome—that is, the successful viable birth of all the fetuses—could be disastrous to the family in financial terms; in practice, it must also be wasteful of scarce and expensive health resources, for no sextuplet is likely to survive without the facilities of the intensive care unit. Equally, the possibility of an emotional catastrophe must be entertained because multiplicity of pregnancy and immaturity of the neonates go hand in hand; thus, the progressive loss of several babies after a prolonged and disturbing struggle to become pregnant must be rated among the greatest tragedies manufactured by modern technology.[19] This brings one to the clinical perspective and the goal of successful motherhood for an apparently infertile woman; the logical solution to the contradictions of superfetation to achieve pregnancy, and limitation of gestations in the quest for viability, is to practise selective reduction of pregnancy—a process which, currently, involves feticide but might, in the relatively near future, be refined into something approaching embryocide.

The moral issues here are almost overwhelming. Fundamentally, the concept of the sanctity of life applies to all the fetuses or *in vivo* embryos involved in a multiple pregnancy as much as it does to the single candidate for abortion or to the several unwanted embryos left *in vitro*. And, if it be argued that the pregnancy is artificial and is, therefore, subject to unnatural manipulation, it is, equally, counter-arguable that this is, of itself, a condemnation of the whole *in vitro* fertilisation programme. The proponent of selective reduction might well introduce the analogy of the overloaded lifeboat—it is better that some, rather than all, should die. But the moral dilemma of the lifeboat has never been solved satisfactorily[20] and, in this scenario, the occupants of the lifeboat are not there through shared misfortune but, rather, as a result of a deliberate act on the part of the authority who will, ultimately, decide their fates, a decision that could be based on such relatively unacceptable criteria as eugenic superiority or, even, sex.

Quite apart from moral considerations, the legality of selective reduction under the terms of the Abortion Act 1967 has to be questioned. Certainly, rearing large numbers of children would be likely to affect the pregnant woman's subsequent health, but the voluntary nature of the pregnancy would tend to throw doubt on the validity of this ground for what is, so far as intention is concerned, primarily feticide rather than fetal death occurring secondarily to termination. The introduction of sextuplets into the family must result in some risk to the physical or mental health of that existing family, though pre-existing children are unlikely in the circumstances of *in vitro* fertilisation. Whether there are grounds for legal termination of pregnancy thus depends, primarily, on whether the retained fetuses can be regarded as being 'existing members of the family' or, secondly, on whether there is sufficient likelihood of physical or mental abnormality deriving from prematurity and very low birth weight.[21] The latter would almost certainly provide acceptable grounds for termination within the ambit of good faith. The former might be more difficult to establish in view of the law's reluctance to attribute legal personality to the fetus. Nevertheless, starting with the words of Stephenson LJ in *McKay*:[22]

> To impose a duty [to terminate the life of a fetus] would be to make a further inroad—in addition to that created by the Abortion Act 1967—into the sanctity of human life which would be contrary to public policy . . .

which clearly impute human life to the fetus—it might not be difficult to make out a convincing case. What is still not clear, however, is whether a partial termination of pregnancy, *per se*, is lawful within the terms of the 1967 Act; it is uncertain whether the term 'a pregnancy' as used in s. 1 refers to the general state of pregnancy or to individual fetal/maternal connections. The fact that selective reduction is certainly being practised suggests that the law is, at the least, willing to turn a blind eye to what may be a technical offence but, nonetheless, arguably good medical practice.

The subject is, however, of very great concern to the Voluntary Licensing Authority which operates in the United Kingdom pending statutory control of modern reproductive techniques. The Authority's response to the issue has been to refuse to license the implantation of more than three embryos at any one time.[23] Banning a practice is, however, no way to decide on its inherent morality or legality. Neither are, currently, well established. At the one extreme, there are those who see selective reduction following *in vitro* fertilisation as one of the most disturbing developments of modern medical practice, carrying with it the power to create and destroy human life in conditions of minimal supervision. On the other hand, it can be held that generalisations are unacceptable when they restrict the best treatment of the individual[24] and that superfetation combined, if necessary, with selective reduction may represent the best treatment in special circumstances. This is surely an area which calls for urgent analysis and legislation before the public becomes too concerned; it is, for example, deeply disturbing to see a newspaper of the quality of *The Times* illustrate an article on medical fertility treatments by a cartoon depicting the baby being thrown out with the bath water.[25]

A concluding word may be directed at the process of uterine lavage. In this, an embryo which is naturally produced within the genital tract of a donor is 'washed out' before implantation and is then transferred to the uterus of a recipient. Despite the clinical advantages claimed for this form of treatment, the method seems so close to veterinary practice that there would seem to be good social reasons for banning it. Despite this antipathy, and for reasons which have been discussed under abortion, the removal of a pre-implantation embryo does not appear to be illegal at present; moreover, it certainly does not offend against a sanctity of life principle. Paradoxically, it is probably that form of embryo transfer which carries the least stigma of disrespect for human life.

Conclusions and Recommendations

9. An Overview

The subject of medical ethics now commands a vast literature—the lists of most publishers include several titles which should have a place in a library of medical jurisprudence, and it follows that this book will have broken little new ground. What I have attempted is to concentrate on the specific question of the value of human life as it exists from conception to the grave and to analyse how this affects current medical practice.

I make neither excuse nor apology for regarding abortion as the pivotal issue in this appraisal. There can be no criticism of organisations which seek to undermine the principle of the sanctity of life from a profession which is responsible for the destruction—often for profit—of living human organisms on the grand scale. On the other side of the coin, however, the rejection of the rigid Genevan principle 'to preserve life from the time of conception' does allow doctors considerably greater leeway in their exercise of clinical judgment, and this may be no bad thing. To offer, and to recapitulate on, some examples of the conclusions which flow from this: therapeutic abortion is preferable to its back-street counterpart; some neonates are so badly defective that they *ought* to be allowed to die before they become aware of their condition; the death of General Franco was, to most observers, a nauseating process; and it is often difficult to see the advantage of a few days of life gained from the use of cytotoxic drugs in a bed-ridden and semi-comatose terminal cancer patient.

But despite these considerations, killing another human remains illegal and, although they may try to dismiss those with opposing views as 'moralist groups pursuing their own ends by threatening doctors with criminal prosecution',[1] doctors who advocate and adopt a quality of life approach to medicine have no inherent entitlement to decide for themselves what should be either illegal or immoral. Moreover, it has to be faced that subtle influences from both within and without the profession are working to edge it ever further from an absolutist view of the value of human life.

The major outside pressure stems from the increasing propagation of, and acceptance of, the cult of personhood. This can be expressed in many different ways but a powerful contemporary philosophy demands, in essence, that, to be a person and to be respected as such, the individual must demonstrate self-awareness and a capacity to make intelligent, even if idiosyncratic, choices.[2] The debate as to 'what is a

105

person?' is one which arises with increasing frequency in medical juris-
prudential debates. In true Socratic style it generates a further analytical
probe: what is the purpose behind the question? Deep down (and it is
fair to describe it as being what is popularly known as 'a gut feeling') we
all know what a person is. It is someone, or a primitive someone, whom
we can recognise as human—some being who is identifiable as either a
male or a female of the human race. Definitions of 'person' in terms of
intellectual criteria are not, therefore, intended to distribute more
widely the rights of and respect for human beings but, rather, are
developed so as to *deprive* some members of the race of such advantages.
Thus, at one end of the life-scale, we have an observer describing
hydrocephalic infants in a special nursery as 'these unfortunate organisms' and going on to say:

> I cannot make myself believe that these unconscious vegetables in
> our hospitals are in any real sense humans . . . Pigeons have more
> personality than this unfortunate moon-calf in our midst.[3]

The writer of this paper was certainly sympathetic and sensitive to the
implications of what he said; but, clearly, it is not difficult to extrapolate
from the intellectual deficiencies of the mentally subnormal to the
incapacity for self-expression which is inherent in normal infancy, and,
before long, personhood is being denied not only to the fetus but also to
the neonate and, still later, to the infant of indeterminate age.

At the other end of life, it is just as apparent that the demented elderly
do not qualify for 'personhood' in terms of self-awareness and self-
expression and that the philosophical proposition thus puts this large
group at special risk of 'disrespect'. Tooley,[4] who supports the concept
wholeheartedly, has tried to get around this criticism by allowing personhood to those who 'have or have had' the necessary mental attributes,
but the exception seems to be little more than an arbitrary device
developed in the cause of a specific defence and one which has no general
application. I am aware that the whole of this book can be interpreted as
representing a call for caution in executing the planned retreat from the
defence of the sanctity of life but perhaps there is no subject where I
would express my concern more forcibly than over the too-ready acceptance and application of the theory of personhood. As Campbell,[5] who is
a protagonist for quality of life principles and whose views are, therefore,
to be taken especially seriously, has explained: life and death decisions
must not be made by default but as a product of 'due process' of medical
practice.

In addition to such outside pressures on the value of life, there are
others which derive intrinsically from the modern approach to the
provision of health care. Foremost among these must be the all-pervad-
ing scarcity of resources. The only circumstance in which resources
approximate to being fully available is within a free market economy.
Their distribution is, then, governed by an ability to pay—Dives can

have what he wants but Lazarus must make do with the crumbs of medical expertise. This may explain the excellent quality of medicine available in the United States[6] where, in addition, extensive private insurance also plays its part. By contrast, rationing is an unfortunate concomitant of public service and, since it is almost unthinkable that the ideals of the British National Health Service would be discarded after nearly half a century, it is inevitable that some form of productivity evaluation must be brought into clinical decision-making. Pressure to concentrate treatment on those patients who are likely to gain most from it are bound to mount on those in charge, say, of intensive care units or on those who see their hospital beds, which were intended for the care of the acutely ill, being occupied by chronically sick geriatric patients.

The profession of medicine within a nationalised service is also becoming more competitive. It is increasingly important to gain specialist qualifications or to publish the results of one's research at ever decreasing levels of training. The profession has only itself to blame that these should be regarded as the main avenues to advancement but, this accepted, it is again an unpalatable fact that abstract values tend to occupy a secondary place in an intensely practical atmosphere. Stemming directly from this, comes, thirdly, Kennedy's[7] concern that doctors now regard themselves as 'scientist problem-solvers and curers'. The danger is that a problem which is difficult to solve may be rationalised as being a life of unacceptable quality. Criticisms such as these can be ignored only at the risk of a loss of confidence between patient and doctor. They are bound to colour any conclusions drawn from the sanctity or quality of life debate. The intention of the following pages is to summarise the debate and to suggest some answers.

Terminal illness

The least complicated of the situations which call for quality of life considerations is that of terminal illness. By definition, there are no curative decisions to be made and good medical practice lies in the treatment of symptoms, and the moral duty is plain. As Pope Paul VI said,

> The duty of the physician consists more in striving to relieve pain than in prolonging as long as possible, with every available means, a life that is no longer fully human and that is naturally coming to its conclusion.[8]

It is, thus, clear that the doctor may apply a productive/non-productive treatment test and that clinical judgment should prevail unless the dying patient positively seeks active (albeit useless) therapeutic intervention, in which case his wishes must be respected. The sanctity, or holiness, of life is minimalised in proportion to its quantity which, in the terminal case, inexorably approaches nil. Quality of life decisions do not arise, for what is being considered is the quality of death. The law has a theoretical interest in preventing fading lives being further shortened but judicial latitude is wide and a prosecution resulting from well-intentioned terminal care is now almost inconceivable.

The problem, both practical and moral, facing the medical profession in this situation is that of how to make the transition from a sanctity of life to a quality of life ethos while, at the same time, ensuring that the pendulum does not swing too far. There can be no doubt that it is now possible to extend the process of terminal illness far beyond natural boundaries; a halt must be called at some point. But the ethical problem lies in how that halt is called. It is perfectly legitimate for the doctor to ask himself: why should I stop this patient dying in peace? But it is another matter to abandon the concept of the sanctity of life so far as to believe that death should be accelerated for the greater benefit of the living. The danger exists and there is much to be said for the view that: 'to continue to speak of the sanctity of life . . . has at least the advantage that it expresses a presumption in favour of trying to preserve it'.[9] Put even more positively: 'by and large, doctors should maintain the presumption in favour of sustaining life'.[10] This presumption is, surely, essential to the medical ethic. Without it, there is the ever present danger of a drift from the concept of 'the comfort of death' to that of defining 'classes of undesirable persons', which might include the aged and might, then, lead to a change from accepting a patient's right to die to establishing a climate of enforcing a duty to die.[11]

The authors of this latter view perceived it to be an increasingly accepted attitude that the role of the physician is to participate in bringing about the desired outcome of death when the benefits of life are seen as insufficient to justify the burden and cost of care. They went on to suggest that such actions should be proscribed pending much fuller debate. Such a need seems doubtful—the arguments have been put and there are now, surely, few thinking doctors who would deny the futility of prolonging death in cases of terminal illness. The option of palliative treatment is open and one hopes that management will be increasingly undertaken by an adequate and highly motivated hospice system which is based not so much on institutionalisation as on a wide concept of community care.[12] Moreover, it is now perfectly clear that, when necessary, it is legitimate to treat symptoms while, at the same time, employing the doctrine of double effect (see p. 18). What both the patient and the public require is an assurance that each decision is carefully weighed. It is no bad thing that physicians should, metaphorically, 'look over their shoulders' when making decisions such as not to resuscitate. There can be no doubt that clinical decisions are best left in the hands of physicians rather than in the hands of the courts;[13] but, equally, each decision ought to be taken in the light of the question: could I convince a court that this decision was *rightly* taken?—for the view of the courts mirrors the view of the society in which that decision is made.

The distinction to be made between withholding aggressive treatment, or 'passive euthanasia', and active intervention to accelerate death is scarcely relevant to the terminal phase of illness and is better discussed in relation to treatable patients and to those who are incompetent.

Incurable disease

The further the clinical condition of the patient is removed from this relatively simple 'terminal' situation, the more complex becomes the doctor's position when assessing the value of a human life. This is shown most vividly in the case of the patient who has no immediately death-dealing disease but is living a life which could be regarded as intolerable because of the pain and suffering involved. The therapeutic options now fall to a choice between an increasing reliance on double effect, through the use of symptomatic treatment which can, and must be, supplemented by supportive measures, and an acceptance of the patient's ultimate expression of autonomy—that is, making a decision to end his own life. In short, since 'passive' euthanasia is not open, the doctor may be faced squarely with a problem involving voluntary active euthanasia which, in this particular circumstance, is indistinguishable from suicide.

I see no easy answer to the problem of the doctor who is invited to assist in suicide. He may well feel that his patient would be better off dead but, when it comes to providing the means of death, he is essentially being invited to make a social rather than a medical decision; thus, he is in no different position from that of anyone else who is close to the would-be suicide. There may be a case—although it has been debated and rejected many times by both the legal profession and the legislature—for altering the criminal law so as to allow the definition of 'mercy killing' as a variety of homicide. What seems certain is that there is no place for legislation which specifically allows a *doctor* to assist a suicide when so asked. It has been argued, I feel rightly, that a change in the law to this end would inhibit progress in the management of the terminally ill[14] and would threaten the normal doctor/patient relationship. Certainly, legislation would be difficult to apply and would be open to exploitation. There is no logical justification for specifically exonerating doctors in such cases. Given the principle of individual self-determination, there is no reason why an intending suicide should not be helped by a pharmacist, a veterinary surgeon or, indeed, anyone with adequate knowledge—and none of these could claim any special protection. It is concluded that doctors whose conscience dictates that they should aid or counsel a suicide should take their chance with the law as it applies to the community as a whole.

So far, discussion has been confined to 'terminal illness' and 'incurable disease'. This is somewhat simplistic as there are, in addition, relatively rare circumstances in which withdrawal of treatment will accelerate death despite the fact that the patient's underlying condition is not immediately life threatening. Such negation of therapy would be extremely improbable in the absence of discussion with and the consent of the patient; the moral problem is, in effect, one which involves only the incompetent. The doctor might, however, find himself faced with a patient's positive refusal to accept life-prolonging treatment—the rejection of cytotoxic drugs for the treatment of advanced malignant disease is a possible example. He may agree with the patient's decision, although he should be careful to ensure that an early determination to, say, 'face death bravely' represents more than just a mood of the moment. He may, on the other hand, disagree and he is very likely to do so in such an extreme, although somewhat theoretical, situation as being requested by a competent patient to turn off a respirator. Although it could be argued that to fail to do so would be treating the patient against his will, no sophistry could eliminate the intuitive reaction that this would be a matter of positive killing of a creature in being. Such cases should, surely, be subject to judicial review. This opinion holds despite any disenchantment with the American experience of such referals. The legal ambience of the United Kingdom is less complicated than is that of the United States—even if only because it contains less than fifty separate legislatures.

It is possible to formulate a very tenable philosophical theory that there is no moral difference between the withdrawal of treatment and the overtly positive 'lethal injection' when the aim of each is to accelerate death. [15] This is particularly so in the neonatal field and the proposition will be addressd more specifically in that connection. Nonetheless, the law is clear: active euthanasia, whether it be of voluntary or involuntary type, is murder. Repeated attempts to alter the law relating to voluntary active euthanasia have failed and opposition has come not only from religious leaders but also from lawyers and the majority of doctors. Despite the fact that there are signs that the attitudes of the last may be changing, and despite the fact that my reasons are based very largely on an unpopular 'slippery slope' argument, I would hope that the law remains unchanged in this respect. The medical profession should resist what would be a massive encroachment on its traditional ethic should the call for active euthanasia gain greater acceptance.

The incompetent patient

Those incompetents whose heart beat is being maintained by mechanical ventilation must be distinguished from those whose vital functions are self-supporting despite the presence of severe cerebral incapacity and the fact that they are suffering from potentially fatal disease. The reason for making this distinction is essentially practical. In the former group, death may occur, so to speak, 'at the flick of the switch'—the physician may either risk or end the existence of a patient by means of what I believe to be a single positive action. In the latter, the option of active 'non-voluntary' euthanasia is, admittedly, there but, in practice, life and death decisions will be resolved through the policy of selective non-treatment; conditions are relatively undramatic and allow for continuous appraisal over a long period. Both situations demand the application of a productive/non-productive treatment test and both entail value judgments as to the quality of life. But the quality of life of a permanently comatose patient in intensive care is so obviously awful that decision-making is relatively simple.

Ventilator death

There are no clinical, moral or legal contraindications to removing a patient from a ventilator once the diagnosis of brain stem death has been made. In fact, there is very little to disturb even those who are unhappy with that particular method of diagnosing death because their main objection lies in its application to the use of 'beating heart donors' in transplantation therapy. All will be content to accept the fact of death once the heart beat has ceased following disconnection from the machine.

As one who has performed autopsies on many bodies with liquefying brains, I have no doubts as to this method of establishing death. It is, however, important to dissociate the primary motive of certifying death from the secondary objective of organ transplantation. This caveat is especially relevant because a distrust of 'body-snatching' has been deeply established in the public mind, largely through sensational reporting in the media. But, no matter how vocal such fears may become, there is no way in which anyone other than the physician immediately concerned can make a diagnosis of death. That is a professional, technical exercise which is the responsibility of the individual and the only body which can dictate the details of a technical method to that individual is one which is composed of his professional peers. I therefore see no purpose in legislation concerning the diagnosis of death although many other jurisdictions have perceived its need. Of the models which are available I suggest that the one adopted in Canada[16] is the most useful because it emphasises the indissoluble feature of the brain-lungs-heart servo-system. This is to be preferred to other solutions, including those in Australia,[17] which are based on an either/or philosophy—death can be diagnosed either by reference to the cardio-respiratory system or to brain function. I would suggest that any legislation introduced into the United Kingdom should be directed not to establishing the diagnosis of death but to codifying the process of organ transplantation. In this respect, it would be reassuring were it to become a legal requirement that a death certificate be completed and handed to the informant of death before any donor operation was undertaken. Not only would this serve to satisfy the relatives of the deceased but the exercise would also crystallise the mind of the certifying physician.

All parties are on less firm ground when considering the management of the ventilated patient who is not benefiting from treatment but who, at the same time, has not been declared brain stem dead. Clearly, no legislation can cover the whole spectrum of factors involved in a decision to withdraw support. The major problem remaining is whether decisions should stay in the hands of the medical profession or whether the courts should become involved as custodians of the public interest. The answer should be 'no' to the latter alternative, not merely because the American experience has been tried and is, as a result, rapidly moving to confine such decision making to clinical hands. Mainly, the opinion is held because it is wholly illogical to suggest that, while it is a matter of medical expertise to institute a particular therapy, it is an extra-professional function to withdraw that line of treatment. What is then involved is the classic application of a productive/non-productive treatment test. It would be only in the most exceptional circumstances that a doctor so acting could be charged with homicide and, were he to be convicted, it would be on such grounds of such perversity that the verdict would be universally acclaimed. It seems well to let well alone.

The self-supporting incompetent

In my view, the most important conceptual aspect of cerebral competence is that the patient who is not brain dead is not dead. Attempts based on the principle of personhood to extend the definition of death by using such terms as cognitive death[18] seem only to confuse the issue and, worse, to exaggerate public fears. Irrespective of the mental capacity of the patient at the time, killing an incompetent is still murder; on the other hand, the greater the degree of permanent brain damage, the more appropriate becomes the application of the twin doctrines of double-effect and of non-productive treatment.

It has, however, been emphasised in chapter 5 that the doctor managing an incompetent is treading not only a narrow moral path but also one strewn with hazards related to both criminal and civil law. In the United States, great emphasis is placed on previous statements of intent made whilst competent. These are seen as being of great help in deciding what constitutes productive treatment and there have been suggestions that 'declarations relating to possible senile illness in the future' should be introduced in Britain. Such calls are sincerely made in search of a mandate for doctors who 'simply do not know what to do for the best in many instances'.[19] But, again, it is doubtful if such declarations have the value attributed to them. In the first place, there is no certainty that the patient would not have had a change of mind—such a change is frequently seen in the competent patient threatened with death; secondly, the doctor is still confined to an extent by the attitudes of the relatives; and, thirdly, it is at least uncertain whether such declarations significantly alter the doctor's position as to criminal law. If it be agreed that the physician has a duty of care and if, as a result, it is accepted that he can commit murder or manslaughter by omission, the consent of the subject to that omission should, in theory, be irrelevant.

Should the law, then be amended by statute to safeguard the doctor in his practice of selective non-treatment? Again, the answer would seem, on balance, to be no, and this for all the same reasons as have caused the downfall of the various euthanasia Bills: legislation would be extremely difficult to draft and even more difficult to implement, and it would always be open to manipulation by the unscrupulous.

So, as has been questioned in the case of the ventilated patient, should the courts become more involved—particularly, say, when non-treatment involves non-feeding? Once more, the feeling is no, but this time rather more firmly. Judges are not clinicians. When they are required to be, as in the United States, one can almost sense them clutching at straws for direction. Thus, distinctions as to 'invasiveness' have been made between, on the one hand, the reinsertion of a gastrostomy tube, which was regarded as being unduly invasive, and, on the other, reliance on an already created stoma to accept the feeding tube, which was considered to be necessary treatment.[20] There is evidence of a movement from the early view that the 'awesome question' of continuing or withholding potentially life-prolonging treatment is one for the law courts which cannot be granted to any other group—including doctors,[21] to one in which good faith and adequate consultation are regarded as the only requirements to ensure that the physician is acting within the law.[22] The latter position is that which is already held in Britain and it would seem unwise to start any movement against the transatlantic stream.

It is surely better that the medical profession itself should adopt a code of practice which can be seen by the public as being rational and acceptable;[23] to balance this, it would perhaps be salutary for the individual doctor to remind himself occasionally that the decision in R v Adams[24] was one which turned on the facts of a jury case—it did not open the side door to the unfettered practice of euthanasia.

The neonate

The therapeutic option of non-treatment of potentially fatal disease has focused on the neonatal period over the last decade and, in many ways, this particular attention is both logical and morally acceptable. We have seen, for example, that the major ethical problem related to ventilator treatment is not of removal from treatment, which is a matter of technique or clinical expertise, but, of *admission* to intensive care. It is reasonable to extend this concept from treatment to life as a whole. Selective non-treatment of the newborn is simply a matter of deciding whether to admit a severely compromised patient to a future of certain pain and doubtful benefit.

So long as this general premise is kept in mind, the practice of selection of the newborn for treatment is morally acceptable and, indeed, compatible with modern Roman Catholic teaching—that is, of course, subject to judgments being made with the greatest caution. [25] It is, however, the potential extension of non-treatment into the arena of neonaticide which is disturbing. The particular importance of such escalation in the neonatal period derives from the inevitable association of death in this early phase of life with abortion. The grounds for abortion have incontrovertibly been extended during twenty years of its legal practice. It is, for example, now unarguable that miscarriages are being procured on non-medical grounds such as the unwanted sex of the fetus. [26] If the role of 'personhood' is accepted as eliding any distinction between the fetus and the neonate, and if, as a result, neonaticide is regarded as an acceptable extension of feticide, then the erosion of the grounds for abortion will be extended to include those for rejection of the newborn—at its extreme, abortion on demand would lead logically to neonaticide on demand. Nowhere is this more evident than in relation to the mentally subnormal infant. If eminent doctors can say: 'in cases [of Down's syndrome] food and water will be withheld in the hopes that complications will develop which will lead to death by natural causes' or, if it can be given in evidence that: 'it is ethical that a child suffering from Down's syndrome . . . should not survive', [27] then it is clear that the movement is well advanced.

It is probable, however, that *Arthur*, rather than making new law or opening the way to widespread neonatal euthanasia, has, paradoxically, served to restrict the application to the newborn infant of a quality of life test. The change of emphasis in the pronouncements of the British Medical Association was marked in the months following the trial and it is probable that this was due at least in part to the opposiition which was voiced by a large proportion of the profession. Later legal analyses of the case have also made it clear that, irrespective of whether Dr Arthur was not guilty, the intentional shortening of a physically healthy child's life by non-feeding must be murder when the regime is prescribed by those with a duty of care for the child. [28]

The moral significance attached to such a basic humane act as providing nourishment for a physically healthy child appears so self-evident that a recapitulation of the omission/commission debate as to culpability in withholding it seems sterile. I would suggest, however, that should any justification be required, neither writing hospital notes nor completing a prescription form for sedative drugs can conceivably be omissions—they must be positive acts which, in the present context, are performed with death in view. Not only does most of the profession recoil from starving a Down's syndrome baby but there is also a wide appreciation that a future Dr Arthur may not be so fortunate in his pathologists.

British law regarding the management of Down's syndrome is, I believe, to be found in *Re B*—not in *Arthur*. The major significance of *Arthur* was that it caused the medical profession to stand still and appraise the direction in which it was going. It seems, now, very unlikely that the precise management schedule which was adopted in the *Arthur* case will be repeated in the United Kingdom in the forseeable future.

Nonetheless, having agreed that there are some *physically* damaged neonates who should not be admitted to intensive treatment, it must, equally, be admitted that there will be grey areas in which the paediatrician may feel concerned about his position. While it is doubtful that such uncertainty will result in a retreat to 'defensive medicine',[29] a situation which leaves room for disquiet is unlikely to encourage a satisfactory clinical atmosphere. 'When human life is at stake, the law . . . should define as precisely as possible the minimal limits which our society considers acceptable'.[30] There does seem to be a good case for legislating to this end in the particular field of neonatal medicine and I have suggested a model elsewhere[31] which runs:

> In the event of positive treatment being necessary for a neonate's survival, it will not be an offence to withhold such treatment if two doctors, one of whom is a consultant paediatrician, acting in good faith and with the consent of both parents if available, decide against treatment in the light of a reasonably clear medical prognosis which indicates that the infant's further life would be intolerable by virtue of pain or suffering or because of severe cerebral incompetence.

This is not creating a new offence through which to confine doctors. It is, admittedly, restrictive, but it is, at the same time, enabling. More importantly, it is directed at the best interests of the infant alone. This situation is so close to abortion that any proposed legislation must be something other than an extension of the Abortion Act 1967 which shows such strong sympathy for the competing rights of the family. Open-ended legislation such as the above must, however be backed by a code of practice, or a framework of acceptable standards for decision-making.[32] With the help of colleagues, I have attempted to formulate such a code, having particular concern to produce a protocol which would be acceptable on both sides of the Atlantic,[33] since international consensus offers a valuable source of reassurance to the public. Our agreed version runs as follows.

If positive treatment is necessary for the infant's survival, the law should respect parental decisions not to treat their newborn when:

1. the decision is concurred in as being medically proper by the attending physician and by at least one other independent, qualified physician, preferably a neonatologist or paediatrician;

2. the medical reasons for the decision not to treat (the prognosis) are entered in the medical record by the physician and are

concurred in by the consultant;

3. the parents have been fully informed of the infant's diagnosis and prognosis with and without any reasonably available treatment; of the risk, nature and benefits of each such treatment; and of any other material facts bearing on the infant's condition and the treatment/non-treatment decision, so that they may give, or refuse, an information-based consent. The explanation and their decision should be likewise entered in the case notes and be witnessed;

4. the judgments required of parents and physicians have been made in good faith with the best interests of the infant as the guiding principle;

5. such affirmative treatment has, when necessary, continued after birth until a clear prognosis can be given with reasonable medical certainty that the infant falls within one of the categories set out below:

(a) that death is highly probable and is expected within a reasonably short time, say one year, regardless of treatment; or

(b) that there is no reasonable possibility that the infant will be able to participate to any degree in human relationships or experiences with others requiring some interaction or response; or

(c) that treatment cannot obviate or alleviate an intolerable level of chronic pain which would make continued life-sustaining treatment inhumane.

We also recommend that manual feeding, not involving medical intervention, should be continued in any circumstances when the infant is capable of taking nourishment by mouth.

Although these guidelines were evolved entirely independently, it is surprising how similar they are to those suggested by Gostin[34] in his major survey of the American position and by the President's Commission on Biomedical Ethics.[35]

If these principles are agreed, the major outstanding question then lies within the killing or letting die controversy. Kuhse,[36] as noted in chapter 6, has argued that there is no moral—or legal—distinction to be made between passivity and activity in the field of neonatal euthanasia. It is, indeed, extremely difficult to fault such an argument logically and, if she is right, it follows inevitably that a quick, controlled death is likely to be less stressful to the infant subject (and, incidentally, to those responsible for it) than is a lingering and uncertain death from natural causes. Yet, quite apart from the manifest illegality of killing a newborn patient, it remains true that there is an intuitive abhorrence of killing, and an intuitive basis of morality is currently receiving a more sympathetic hearing than it has been afforded in the past.[37] In addition, few paediatricians would wish to take on the mantle of executioner. In the end, it is difficult to improve on the intuitive position adopted by the President of the British Paediatric Association who wrote:

The very great majority of paediatricians, while accepting the practice of abortion when severe fetal abnormalities can be detected in early pregnancy, do not countenance the deliberate killing of a deformed new-born baby who, with ordinary care, would survive. Thus we are guilty of inconsistency but not of infanticide . . .[38]
Put another way, this may be a situation where the best that can be said is that the kindest course is, unfortunately, not that which is most morally acceptable.

But it is still difficult to dismiss the 'slippery slope' argument entirely. It is not a great step for a profession which embraces feticide to accept active neonaticide and this is, surely, a potential gradation which should be strongly resisted. It is easily and very widely held that once abortion is accepted with only minor restrictions, so there should be no greater objection to killing the neonate. Perhaps Ramsey's reverse view[39] that, if killing the neonate is legally unacceptable, then so also should be the killing of a fetus, deserves more consideration than it is generally given.

Abortion

The centrality of abortion to the sanctity of life debate has been emphasised throughout this book. Whether or not this interpretation is accepted depends, at the extremes, on whether or not the fetus is believed to be a human being, albeit an immature one, or whether it is regarded as an occasional product of sexual intercourse to be retained or disposed of at its mother's behest. The near impossibility of defining when human life begins is fully admitted but it is suggested that to adopt a policy of 'gradualism' is not only to beg the question but, at the same time, to introduce unacceptable uncertainties. The decision has to be made of choosing some recognisable point lying between conception and, say, late childhood. My firm conclusion is to regard implantation as the critical point at which humanity is acquired and at which respect as a human being becomes due.

It follows that I believe abortion to be the taking of human life and that, therefore, it is an act for which there can be no overall condonation. A philosophical theory which places contraception and abortion on the same moral plane cannot be maintained once implantation is accepted as representing the watershed of humanity—nor, in particular, can those theories be accepted which attempt to justify abortion as a legitimate form of population control or as a means of reducing the number of unwanted children.[40] The number of infertile women anxious for a family is not grossly disproportionate to the number of fertile women who wish to terminate their pregnancy. Feticide and, to a lesser extent, neonaticide could be largely balanced by adoption which would, in passing, serve also to reduce the need for the production of and destruction of embryos. It is undeniable that the effects of the pregnancy itself, rather than those of motherhood, will constitute the grounds for termination in a large proportion of cases, and it would be quite unacceptable to force gestation and labour upon a woman who, otherwise, qualifies for a legal termination of pregnancy; yet one wonders what proportion of women seeking such relief receive active counselling as to the possibility of adoption—and, even more, what positive steps governments are prepared to take to promote adoption as a preferred alternative.

But to take such a stance is not necessarily to be absolutist. Indeed, the root of the difficulties and misunderstandings encountered in this area lies in the entrenched polarisation of extreme positions. On the one hand, we have increasingly strident calls to abandon respect for the fetus in favour of an absolute right of women to repudiate what is, perhaps unfortunately, a matter of the natural order of human sexuality; on the other, we have the unattractive example of people praying for the death of a judge so that he may be replaced by one of a different moral persuasion.[41] It becomes hard at times to decide who is the more difficult to love—the radical feminist or the religious bigot.

It is even more sad that the abortion issue has been taken up as a matter of party politics. Without doubt, the most distasteful piece of political propaganda I have seen is a poster depicting a pregnant woman; her fetus *in utero* sports a Reagan button while she wears one favouring Mr Mondale. Our academic and professional leaders emerge little better. Thus, we have a contributor to the *Journal of Medical Ethics* writing:

> the war against abortion is well and truly on. Its political impli-
> cations as America moves further and further to the Right are
> frightening . . .[42]

while, in Britain, the call for 'abortion on demand' has become a standard political plank of the far left.

The number of abortions has climbed at an almost steady rate to reach approximately 170 per cent of the 1970 figure in both England and Wales and in Scotland so that there were over 182 000 abortions in Great Britain in 1986. It is possible to see this as a thoroughly practical solution to an unfortunate problem but, surely, no one can be *happy* in such a situation.

Given current attitudes to sexual intercourse, the most obvious way to limit the increase in controversial abortions is to improve contraceptive facilities. It may well be that both processes are designed to limit the number of unwanted children but, *pace* Jonathan Glover, I cannot see contraceptive services reflecting the *value* of human life. A moral distinction between contraception and abortion becomes particularly obvious when one looks at the case of *Gillick*.[43] It is surely self-evident that teenage contraception is to be distinguished from and is, at least, less undesirable than teenage abortion. Contraception may *prevent* human life; it certainly does not *destroy* it and the process does not involve surgical trauma. The relationship between the two—and, indeed, between them and sexual moderation—is an interesting and complicated subject but I see it as being beyond the scope of my title.

Rather, the challenge must be to devise some check on current trends while finding common ground between the opposing claims of women and the unborn within the current social and legal ambience. As a starting point, it has to be accepted that the concept of relatively easy therapeutic abortion has been with us for twenty years and is here to stay. Nevertheless, we are, at the same time, witnessing an increase in the appreciation of fetal rights, although this movement is firmly tied to the concept of increasing respect for the fetus *pari passu* with its increasing maturity. Thus, as things stand at present, the fetus attracts a status comparable to that of its mother when it becomes viable.[44] Viability, however, is a nebulous idea (see p.76). If a finite point is needed at which the fetus is to be granted a right to life, it would be better fixed at that point when it is 'capable of being born alive'.[45] This preference derives from the fact that a live-born neonate is entitled to a birth certificate irrespective of its capacity to survive.

Until recently, the definition of a live birth was in some dispute. The only indication available under United Kingdom statute law came from assuming the contrary of the definition of a stillbirth[46]—which would mean that a child which 'breathed or showed any other sign of life after being fully separated from its mother' was born alive.[47] It is the words 'any other sign of life' which have caused difficulty. Williams, for example, has held that the test of 'living' lies in the functioning of the heart,[47] and, in this, he has the support of the World Health Organisation who include 'beating of the heart' as evidence that the product of a birth is 'live born'. I submit that this could never have been so. In the first place, it would have meant that virtually any miscarriage other than that of a macerated fetus after about the eighteenth week of pregnancy would constitute a live birth. Secondly, it would, in practice, have made a mockery of any intent to distinguish pathologically between live and still birth—indeed, it would be frankly impossible to do so on the basis of the presence of a heart beat.

The matter has now been put beyond doubt in England in 1987 by the decision in C v S[48] in which a live birth was defined in terms of an ability to breathe with or without assistance of a ventilator. Such a status is unlikely to be reached before the twenty-fourth week of gestation. The Abortion (Amendment) Bill 1987 is still being debated at the time of writing and it is not known whether the modest measures deriving from the ill-fated Infant Life (Preservation) Bill 1987 (see p.83) will be accepted; these had the general support of those professionals most closely involved in the performance of therapeutic abortions.[49] Nonetheless, there are now some ground rules on which we can draw.

Twenty-four weeks can be taken as that point at which the fetus should attain maximum respect and it seems quite wrong that doctors terminating a pregnancy at or about that time should feel compelled by law to manage the operation so as to ensure a stillborn abortus. Rather, it is logical to hold that a therapeutic abortion of a fetus of more than, say, twenty-two weeks' gestation should be performed in conditions which are designed, so far as possible, to assist the potentially viable abortus to survive. Such measures might require legislation and, admittedly, this would be difficult to frame so as to ensure that it took in adequately the possibility of neonatal or infantile disease which was due solely to prematurity. I would suggest an inserted clause in the 1967 Act on the following lines:

A termination of pregnancy involving a fetus which is likely to be capable of attaining a separate existence is to be carried out, save in an emergency to preserve the life of the mother, with the intention of assisting the abortus to live. In applying treatment to this end, the doctor may take into account the actual physical state of the infant and also the forseeable effect of prematurity on its future development.

Subject to the mother's agreement, a fetus so saved is to be regarded as an abandoned child and may be offered for adoption.

At the other end of the 'fetal maturity' scale, we have the conceptus or zygote which, by analogy, must have minimal rights vis à vis its mother. It now seems to me that there is a case for abandoning the stance that all terminations of pregnancy which are performed at a very early period of gestation are justified by strict clinical criteria. Accordingly, it might be more honest to admit to abortion at the request of a woman. Quite what should be the length of this 'permissive period' is not easy to say. Pragmatically, twelve weeks' gestation, or the mid-point between minimum and maximum fetal rights, seems reasonable. The essential corollary to such a change in legal attitudes would be that the grounds for therapeutic abortion between twelve and twenty-four weeks' gestation should take progressively greater account of fetal interests when assessing the maternal/fetal balance. A simple way to do this would be to insert the pre-condition that the continuation of the pregnancy would have a '*grave* effect on the health of the mother'. This was a feature—albeit intended for application throughout pregnancy—of the unsuccessful Abortion (Amendment) Bill 1979.

Modifications of this nature would not be revolutionary; they would bring United Kingdom law closer to that of the United States and very similar to that accepted in many other jurisdictions including countries in the Eastern European Communist bloc.

It could, of course, be claimed that a 'three tiered' approach to abortion would be difficult to understand, difficult to apply and invasive of the doctor's clinical independence. Nevertheless, the proposals represent an attempt at rationalising the position by giving ground to both parties who are, unfortunately, becoming identified as the 'pro-choice' and 'pro-life' lobbies. Moreover, there are still many doctors who see the

Abortion Act as a massive interference with the fundamentals of medical ethics. It is, in fact, my main ground for disagreement with those who support 'abortion on demand' that, in so doing, they impose an unsolicited obligation on the medical profession. A case can, indeed, be made for excluding a doctor/patient relationship from abortions which have no therapeutic dimension; there is no reason why 'terminations of convenience', if permitted, should not be performed by trained abortionists.

My suggestions are, however, subject to the more fundamental objection that they are inconsistent when judged by my own standards. Given that humanity is bestowed at implantation, the deliberate procurement of *any* miscarriage carries with it the same potential moral stigma irrespective of the gestational maturity of the abortus. This criticism is very valid. The proposals as set out are justifiable only on doubtful utilitarian grounds—they represent an effort to please the greatest number of persons. Were I to be asked to carry out a 'demand' abortion in the first twelve weeks of pregnancy I admit that I would claim the privilege of conscience,[50] but this is no more than a confession of an inability to provide a reasoned justification for what could be looked upon as no better than bowing to reality.

I would also argue very strongly for a modification of the Act so that the 'fetal grounds' for abortion were clearly expressed as being directed to the interests of the fetus rather than of the mother. The reasons for this are several although the most important refer, directly or indirectly, to respect for the status of the fetus. Conceptually, we have returned to the close relationship that exists between abortion and neonaticide. I have argued at length that neonaticide, which would include selective non-treatment of the newborn, is morally and legally acceptable only when it is practised for the benefit of the infant—indeed, this is the basic reason why parental rights to reject their child, if there are such rights, must be closely supervised. Once it is accepted that, save in circumstances controlled by deep religious conviction, those infants who are selected for non-treatment would have been aborted had they been diagnosed *in utero*, it follows that it is illogical to regard the legality of such an abortion as being grounded in maternal interests. To maintain such an attitude means either that infanticide, using the word in the legal sense and extending it to the parents rather than limiting it to the mother only, should not only be decriminalised, but should be positively condoned; and, if this is regarded as unacceptable, as it must be, then Ramsey's hypothesis[51] (see p.117) is fully vindicated and abortion should not be allowed.

Attitudes to abortion on behalf of the fetus are, admittedly, often opposed. Brahams, for example, positively criticises the Abortion Act 1967, s.(1)(1)(b) for discriminating between a normal and a handicapped fetus where the latter is, by inference reduced to the status of a disposable commodity.[52] On the other side, there are those who, like myself, regard the fetal reasons as being the most acceptable grounds for abortion other than those for actually saving the life of the mother. This, again, is based on the interests of the fetus which receive scant notice in most legislations. Thus, we have already seen that the legality of abortion performed for fetal reasons is doubtful even in those Australian States which take a liberal approach to abortion and, although the point has not, to my knowledge, been tested, the combination of the time taken to undertake genetic screening and the absence of a specific opinion on the matter in Roe v Wade[53] may force many 'eugenic' abortions in the United States into the illegal category.[54]

I would therefore hope to see the position clarified in Great Britain and to have the 'fetal grounds' detached from the 'maternal grounds' in defining a legal abortion. This would involve adding to the 'fetal clause' (s.1(1)(b)) a phrase such as: 'and that, as a result, its quality of life would be severely compromised'.[55] A main theoretical advantage of a clear separation of that type is that it would eliminate the inequity which is inherent in the judgment in McKay[56] (see p.80). It seems indefensible to allow the mother grounds for abortion because she would otherwise be encumbered by a defective child—and, hence, to have grounds for an action in tort when negligently deprived of that opportunity—and yet, at the same time, to deny the fetus a right to say that his congenital disabilities are such that he would prefer to have nothing more to do with life. The competent adult is entitled to refuse treatment and the neonate is offered a similar de facto, if not de jure, opportunity. Why, then, should the fetus be denied this expression of autonomy? A clear transfer of interest would also settle the difficult question of the 'wrongful life' action. Currently, a defective child who is born because of negligent counselling of its mother has no right of action against the counsellor because the latter was not responsible for, or the cause of, the disability. Problems of causation are, however, minimised in the suggested revised legislation under which the fetus could claim that it was he who was wrongly informed and who was, thus, deprived of a choice.[57]

The second, and perhaps more practical, advantage of distinguishing what Ramsey has called 'fetal euthanasia' from abortion is that the separation could be used to eliminate the current conflict between, on the one hand, the provision of adequate genetic screening and, on the other, the possible commission of the English crime of child destruction.[58] I have already set out the logical argument for protecting the life of a 24-week-old fetus as being that of one which is capable of a separate existence. As things stand, adequate investigations for severe genetic abnormality may not be completed within that time and it would be an essential corollary to exempt the fetus who is acting in his own interests from such a time limitation.[59] It should be reiterated that this particular difficulty is likely to evaporate as new techniques, including that of chorionic villus sampling, are developed. Nonetheless, the law should be clear.

I am conscious that these proposals will almost certainly be misinterpreted. It is clear from my views on the attribution of humanity that I cannot approve of abortion 'on demand' or for 'convenience'. Abortion is, to my mind, the taking of human life, and to argue that it is inferior life and, therefore, an inferior offence is not far from saying that to murder an alcoholic outcast is less of an offence than to murder a bishop. I cannot empathise with the 'pro-choice' movement because, as Callahan has pointed out,[60] in defining the issue as one of absolute rights the movement has never made sufficient room in its public stance for a consideration of the fetus. Similarly, any suggestion that it is reprehensible to be born with a congenital defect is abhorrent.

The answers to these problems lie, firstly, in responsible attitudes to sexual intercourse and contraception and, secondly, in a massive improvement of institutional and adoptive care facilities for the handicapped. But to weep for such objectives in a pluralistic and economically vulnerable society is to cry for the moon. We have to live in the world as it is and not as we would like it to be. My proposals are essentially a compromise, the purpose of which is to counter the self-interested approach to abortion which is evolving and to set a limit to this particular form of devaluation of human life. The tide may, indeed, be turning.[61]

Embryocide

There seems little point in equivocation over the status of, and the management of, the *in vitro* embryo—either the embryo is a human being or it is not. I believe that it is not, this opinion being based on the presumption that humanity derives from human contact. This is not to deny that the embryo is certainly human tissue and is, therefore, not to be treated with total disrespect—and this underlies the reason why the deliberate production of embryos for the purpose of research and experimentation is to be deprecated.

I wonder why, in fact, there is so much emotion associated with the disposal of embryos when so little concern is shown for the fetus. Perhaps it is no more than a matter of cynical politics? A stance on the abortion issue is electorally neutral; comparable support will come from either the 'pro-life' or the 'pro-choice' constituency, depending on which way the politician faces. Opposition to any form of embryocide will, however, gather support from the former, while the 'pro-choice' lobby will remain emotionally uninvolved—a net gain in popularity is thus likely. It is, fairer to suppose that politicians see *in vitro* fertilisation as a new technique which certainly has frightening possibilities. As I write this, the Vatican has issued a statement condemning the practice of *in vitro* fertilisation. The grounds for this may be arguable[62] but it does show a firm commitment to consistency across the continuum of embryocide, feticide and neonaticide.

Conclusion

Developments in medicine *can* be disturbing. There is no doubt that changes in medical thinking have evolved over the last half century and, among these, the acceptance of death as an option in therapeutic intention plays a significant role. Moreoever, any rejection of the fundamental vow to maintain the utmost respect for human life from the moment of conception now has strong legislative support in the form of the Abortion Act 1967.

It is, of course, proper that declarations of principle should be adaptable to changing times but there is always a danger of an unconscious drift beyond the intended limits; the spectre of lives being in danger when they become a burden to their fellow men[63] is not entirely a figment of science fiction. Abortion is the propellant of any movement away from Hippocratic principles and, in only a few years, all active medical practitioners will have trained in hospitals in which the juxtaposition of the abortion clinic and the paediatric intensive care unit is regarded as normal.

Perhaps both the medical and legal professions—and the general public—should be hesitant before dismissing out of hand those who still fight for the sanctity of *all* human life. The anti-abortion, 'pro-life', organisations on both sides of the Atlantic may do, and have done, some ill-advised things but it may not be true that they 'know very little of the virtue of compassion'.[64] Their intransigence can be exasperating but it is just possible that, in the long run, they may turn out to be major custodians of the human conscience.

Appendix A*

OFFENCES AGAINST THE PERSON ACT 1861
(24 & 25 Vict c 100)

Attempts to procure Abortion

58 Administering drugs or using instruments to procure abortion
Every woman, being with child, who, with intent to procure her own miscarriage, shall unlawfully administer to herself any poison or other noxious thing, or shall unlawfully use any instrument or other means whatsoever with the like intent, and whosoever, with intent to procure the miscarriage of any woman, whether she be or be not with child, shall unlawfully administer to her or cause to be taken by her any poison or other noxious thing, or shall unlawfully use any instrument or other means whatsoever with the like intent, shall be guilty of felony, and being convicted thereof shall be liable . . . to be kept in penal servitude for life . . .

59 Procuring drugs, etc, to cause abortion
Whosoever shall unlawfully supply or procure any poison or other noxious thing, or any instrument or thing whatsoever, knowing that the same is intended to be unlawfully used or employed with intent to procure the miscarriage of any woman, whether she be or be not with child, shall be guilty of a misdemeanor, and being convicted thereof shall be liable . . . to be kept in penal servitude . . .

---

* The texts of these Statutes are as given in Halsbury's Statutes, 4th edition, Vol. 12 (with occasional Scottish additions).

Appendix B

INFANT LIFE (PRESERVATION) ACT 1929
(19 & 20 Geo 5 c 34)

An Act to amend the law with regard to the destruction of children at or before birth [10 May 1929]

Northern Ireland. This Act does not apply; see s.3(2) post.

1 Punishment for child destruction

(1) Subject as hereinafter in this subsection provided, any person who, with intent to destroy the life of a child capable of being born alive, by any wilful act causes a child to die before it has an existence independent of its mother, shall be guilty of felony, to wit, of child destruction, and shall be liable on conviction thereof on indictment to penal servitude for life:

Provided that no person shall be found guilty of an offence under this section unless it is proved that the act which caused the death of the child was not done in good faith for the purpose only of preserving the life of the mother.

(2) For the purposes of this Act, evidence that a woman had at any material time been pregnant for a period of twenty-eight weeks or more shall be prima facie proof that she was at that time pregnant of a child capable of being born alive.

2 Prosecution of offences

(1) . . .

(2) Where upon the trial of any person for the murder or manslaughter of any child, or for infanticide, or for an offence under section fifty-eight of the Offences against the Person Act 1861 (which relates to administering drugs or using instruments to procure abortion), the jury are of opinion that the person charged is not guilty of murder, manslaughter or infanticide, or of an offence under the said section fifty-eight, as the case may be, but that he is shown by the evidence to be guilty of the felony of child destruction, the jury may find him guilty of that felony, and thereupon the person convicted shall be liable to be punished as if he had been convicted upon an indictment for child destruction.

(3) Where upon the trial of any person for the felony of child

126

destruction the jury are of opinion that the person charged is not guilty of that felony, but he is shown by the evidence to be guilty of an offence under the said section fifty-eight of the Offences against the Person Act 1861, the jury may find him guilty of that offence, and thereupon the person convicted shall be liable to be punished as if he had been convicted upon an indictment under that section.

(4) . . .

(5) *Section four of the Criminal Evidence Act 1898 shall have effect as if this Act were included in the schedule to that Act.*

3 Short title and extent

(1) This Act may be cited as the Infant Life (Preservation) Act 1929.

(2) This Act shall not extend to Scotland or Northern Ireland.

Appendix C

SUICIDE ACT 1961
(9 & 10 Eliz 2 c 60)

An Act to amend the law of England and Wales relating to suicide, and for purposes connected therewith [3 August 1961]

1 Suicide to cease to be a crime
The rule of law whereby it is a crime for a person to commit suicide is hereby abrogated.

2 Criminal liability for complicity in another's suicide
(1) A person who aids, abets, counsels or procures the suicide of another, or an attempt by another to commit suicide, shall be liable on conviction on indictment to imprisonment for a term not exceeding fourteen years.

(2) If on the trial of an indictment for murder or manslaughter it is proved that the accused aided, abetted, counselled or procured the suicide of the person in question, the jury may find him guilty of that offence.

(3) The enactments mentioned in the first column of the First Schedule to this Act shall have effect subject to the amendments provided for in the second column (which preserve in relation to offences under ths section the previous operation of those enactments in relation to murder or manslaughter).

(4) . . . no proceedings shall be instituted for an offence under this section except by or with the consent of the Director of Public Prosecutions.

3 Short title, repeal and extent
(1) This Act may be cited as the Suicide Act 1961.

(2) . . .

(3) This Act shall extend to England and Wales only, except as regards the amendments made by Part II of the First Schedule and except that the Interments (felo de se) Act 1882 shall be repealed also for the Channel Islands.

Appendix D

ABORTION ACT 1967
(1967 c 87)

An Act to amend and clarify the law relating to termination of pregnancy by registered medical practitioners   [27 October 1967]

1 Medical termination of pregnancy

(1) Subject to the provisions of ths section, a person shall not be guilty of an offence under the law relating to abortion when a pregnancy is terminated by a registered medical practitioner if two registered medical practitioners are of the opinion, formed in good faith—

(a) that the continuance of the pregnancy would involve risk to the life of the pregnant woman, or of injury to the physical or mental health of the pregnant woman or any existing children of her family, greater than if the pregnancy were terminated; or

(b) that there is a substantial risk that if the child were born it would suffer from such physical or mental abnormalities as to be seriously handicapped.

(2) In determining whether the continuance of a pregnancy would involve such risk of injury to health as is mentioned in paragraph (a) of subsection (1) of this section, account may be taken of the pregnant woman's actual or reasonably foreseeable environment.

(3) Except as provided by subsection (4) of this section, any treatment for the termination of pregnancy must be carried out in a hospital vested in [the Secretary of State for the purposes of his functions under the National Health Service Act 1977 or the National Health Service (Scotland) Act 1978 or in a place approved for the purposes of this section by the Secretary of State].

(4) Subsection (3) of this section, and so much of subsection (1) as relates to the opinion of two registered medical practitioners, shall not apply to the termination of a pregnancy by a registered medical practitioner in a case where he is of the opinion, formed in good faith, that the termination is immediately necessary to save the life or to prevent grave permanent injury to the physical or mental health of the pregnant woman.

2 Notification

(1) The [Secretary of State] in respect of England and Wales, and the Secretary of State in respect of Scotland, shall by statutory instrument make regulations to provide—

(a) for requiring any such opinion as is referred to in section 1 of this Act to be certified by the practitioners or practitioner concerned in such form and at such time as may be prescribed by the regulations, and for requiring the preservation and disposal of certificates made for the purposes of the regulations;

(b) for requiring any registered medical practitioner who terminates a pregnancy to give notice of the termination and such other information relating to the termination as may be so prescribed;

(c) for prohibiting the disclosure, except to such persons or for such purposes as may be so prescribed, of notices given or information furnished pursuant to the regulations.

(2) The information furnished in pursuance of regulations made by virtue of paragraph (b) of subsection (1) of this section shall be notified solely to the [Chief Medical Officer of the Department of Health and Social Security, or of the Welsh Office, or of the Scottish Home and Health Department].

(3) Any person who wilfully contravenes or wilfully fails to comply with the requirements of regulations under subsection (1) of this section shall be liable on summary conviction to a fine not exceeding [level 5 on the standard scale].

(4) Any statutory instrument made by virtue of this section shall be subject to annulment in pursuance of a resolution of either House of Parliament.

3 Application of Act to visiting forces etc

(1) In relation to the termination of a pregnancy in a case where the following conditions are satisfied, that is to say—

(a) the treatment for termination of the pregnancy was carried out in a hospital controlled by the proper authorities of a body to which this section applies; and

(b) the pregnant woman had at the time of the treatment a relevant association with that body; and

(c) the treatment was carried out by a registered medical practitioner or a person who at the time of the treatment was a member of that body appointed as a medical practitioner for that body by the proper authorities of that body,

this Act shall have effect as if any reference in section 1 to a registered medical practitioner and to a hospital vested in [the Secretary of State] included respectively a reference to such a person as is mentioned in paragraph (c) of this subsection and to a hospital controlled as aforesaid, and as if section 2 were omitted.

(2) The bodies to which this section applies are any force which is a visiting force within the meaning of any of the provisions of Part I of the Visiting Forces Act 1952 and any headquarters within the meaning of the Schedule to the International Headquarters Defence Organisations Act 1964; and for the purposes of this section—

(a) a woman shall be treated as having a relevant association at any time with a body to which this section applies if at that time—

(i) in the case of such a force as aforesaid, she had a relevant association within the meaning of the said Part I with the force; and

(ii) in the case of such headquarters as aforesaid, she was a member of the headquarters or a dependant within the meaning of the Schedule aforesaid of such a member; and

(b) any reference to a member of a body to which this section applies shall be construed—

(i) in the case of such a force as aforesaid, as a reference to a member of or of a civilian component of that force within the meaning of the said Part I; and

(ii) in the case of such a headquarters as aforesaid, as a reference to a member of that headquarters within the meaning of the Schedule aforesaid.

4 Conscientious objection to participation in treatment

(1) Subject to subsection (2) of this section, no person shall be under any duty, whether by contract or by any statutory or other legal requirement, to participate in any treatment authorised by this Act to which he has a conscientious objection:

Provided that in any legal proceedings the burden of proof of conscientious objection shall rest on the person claiming to rely on it.

(2) Nothing in subsection (1) of this section shall affect any duty to participate in treatment which is necessary to save the life or to prevent grave permanent injury to the physical or mental health of a pregnant woman.

(3) In any proceedings before a court in Scotland, a statement on oath by any person to the effect that he has a conscientious objection to participating in any treatment authorised by this Act shall be sufficient evidence for the purpose of discharging the burden of proof imposed upon him by subjection (1) of this section.

5 Supplementary provisions

(1) Nothing in this Act shall affect the provisions of the Infant Life (Preservation) Act 1929 (protecting the life of the viable foetus).

(2) For the purposes of the law relating to abortion, anything done with intent to procure the miscarriage of a woman is unlawfully done unless authorised by section 1 of this Act.

6 Interpretation

In this Act, the following expressions have meanings hereby assigned to them:—

'the law relating to abortion' means sections 58 and 59 of the Offences against the Person Act 1861, and any rule of law relating to the procurement of abortion;

7 Short title, commencement and extent

(1) This Act may be cited as the Abortion Act 1967.

(2) This Act shall come into force on the expiration of the period of six months beginning with the date on which it is passed.

(3) This Act does not extend to Northern Ireland.

Notes

CHAPTER ONE
A Perspective
1. *War Crimes and Medicine* (1947) Statement by the Council of the Association for Submission to the W.M.A., July 1947, London: BMA House.
2. The texts of the various oaths and declarations quoted are those given in *Dictionary of Medical Ethics* (Revised edn, 1981) Eds. A. S. Duncan, G. R. Dunstan and R. B. Welbourn, London: Darton, Longman and Todd.
3. E. Slater, 'Severely malformed children: Wanted—a new basic approach' |1973| 1 *Brit Med J* 285.
4. J. Lorber, 'Spina bifida cystica. Results of treatment of 270 consecutive cases with criteria for selection for the future' (1972) 47 *Arch Dis Childh* 854.
5. J. Lorber, 'Ethical problems in the management of myelomeningocele and hydrocephalus' (1975) 10 *J. Roy Coll Phycns* 47.
6. R. S. Duffy and A. G. M. Campbell, 'Moral and ethical dilemmas in a special-care nursery' (1973) 289 *New Engl J Med* 890.
7. 'We believe life is not ours. We do not own life to be able to dispose of it and therefore the obligation to preserve life is regarded as a religious precept', I. Jakobovits, Chief Rabbi, quoted by L. Green (1980) 6 *BMA News Rev* (5) 57. See also the valuable review article I. Jakobovits, 'Jewish medical ethics—a brief overview' (1983) 9 *J Med Ethics* 109.
8. S. Jacobson, 'The right to life' (1979) 19 *J Forens Sci Soc* 87.
9. P. Singer, 'Sanctity of life or quality of life?' (1983) 72 *Pediatrics* 128. See also the resulting letters to the Editor (1984) 73 *Pediatrics* 259-61.
10. J. Locke, *Essay Concerning Human Understanding*, Book II, ch.9, para 29; J. Fletcher, 'Indicators of humanhood: A tentative profile of man' (1972) *Hastings Center Report*, No.5.
11. See, for example, J. Cadoux, *The Early Christian Attitude to War* (1919) London: Allen & Unwin quoted in H. Harris, *Pre-natal Diagnosis and Elective Abortion* (1974) London: Nuffield Provincial Hospitals Trust.
12. J. S. Mill, *On Liberty and Representative Government* (1948) London: Blackwell's Political Texts, p.8.
13. See, for instance, the major example in this decade of I. Kennedy, *The Unmasking of Medicine* (1981) London: George Allen & Unwin.
14. J. K. Mason and R. A. McCall Smith, *Law and Medical Ethics* (2nd edn, 1987) London: Butterworths, pp.6 *et seq.*
15. Editorial Comment 'Death without concealment' (1981) 283 *Brit Med J* 1629.
16. This is convincingly argued in the context of the child in W. A. Silverman, 'A hospice setting for human neonatal death' (1982) 69 *Pediatrics* 239.

17. Note that the Declaration of Sydney, published *after* the Abortion Act, interprets life as existing 'from the time of conception'.
18. Editorial Comment 'No case for an Abortion Bill' [1979] 2 *Brit Med J* 230.
19. J. D. J. Havard (1982) 284 *Brit Med J* 612.
20. H. Beynon [1982] Crim L R 17.
21. Quoted by D. Brahams and M. Brahams in 'R *v* Arthur—is legislation appropriate?' (1981) 78 *Law Soc Gaz* 1342.

CHAPTER TWO
Terminal Illness

1. For an expression of this, see the conclusion to the early but outstanding work D. W. Meyers, *The Human Body and the Law* (1970) Edinburgh: University Press, pp.158-9. See also M. Lappé, 'Dying while living: A critique of allowing to die legislation' (1978) 4 *J Med Ethics* 195.
2. R. G. Twycross, 'Euthanasia—a physician's viewpoint' (1982) 8 *J Med Ethics* 86.
3. 368 Parl Deb HL 1976, pp.196-214, 226-9, 249-81.
4. R. A. McCormick, 'To save or let die. The dilemma of modern medicine' (1974) 229 *J Amer Med Ass* 172.
5. I. M. Kennedy, 'The legal definition of death' (1973) 41 *Med-Leg J* 36.
6. Lord Scarman, 'Legal liability and medicine' (1981) 74 *J Roy Soc Med* 11.
7. G. S. Robertson, 'Dealing with the brain-damaged old—dignity before sanctity' (1982) 8 *J Med Ethics* 173. It is fair to say, however, that the author does not approve of ths option.
8. There is a mass of literature on the subject. Excellent reviews are to be found in S. A. M. McLean and A. J. McKay, 'Consent in medical treatment' in S. A. M. McLean (ed.) *Legal Issues in Medicine* (1981) Aldershot: Gower; P. D. G. Skegg, *Law, Ethics and Medicine* (1984) Oxford: Clarendon Press; H. Teff, 'Consent to medical procedures: Paternalism, self-determination or therapeutic alliance?' (1985) 101 LQR 432.
9. In *Sidaway v Bethlem Royal Hospital Governors and others* [1984] 2 WLR 778, CA at p.795.
10. *Bolam v Friern Hospital Management Committee* [1957] 1 WLR 583 approved in *Sidaway*, above, [1985] 2 WLR 480, HL.
11. I. Kennedy, 'The legal effect of requests by the terminally ill and aged not to receive further treatment from doctors' [1976] Crim LR 217.
12. *Superintendent of Belchertown State School v Saikewicz* 370 NE 2d 417 (Mass, 1977).
13. N. L. Cantor, 'Quinlan, privacy, and the handling of incompetent dying patients' (1977) 30 *Rutgers L Rev* 243. See, for example, *Re Quackenbush* 383 A 2d 785 (NJ, 1978).
14. For discussion, see Zellick, n.7, ch.4 below.
15. G. Williams, 'Down's syndrome and the doctor's responsibility' (1981) 131 *NLJ* 1040.
16. For an easy philosophical discussion, see R. Gillon, 'Justice and allocation of medical resources' (1985) 291 *Brit Med J* 266.
17. *Per* Devlin, J. Quoted in H. Palmer, 'Dr Adams' trial for murder' [1957] Crim LR 365.

18. See n.2 above.
19. This is quoted by S. McLean and G. Maher in *Medicine, Morals and the Law*, ch.3, n.12. Father Donaldson also provided me with the same explanation.
20. (1957) 49 *Acta Apostolicae Sedis* 147.
21. Sacred Congregation for the Doctrine of the Faith *Declaration on Euthanasia* (1980) Vatican: Polyglot Press.
22. D. Coggan, 'On dying and dying well—moral and spiritual aspects' (1977) 70 *Proc R Soc Med* 75.
23. *Decisions of Life and Death: A Problem in Modern Medicine* (1965), Board for Social Responsibility of the Church of England, p.50.
24. G. Williams, *The Sanctity of Life and the Criminal Law* (1958) London: Faber and Faber, p.286.
25. N.24 above, p.288.
26. G. Williams, *Textbook of Criminal Law* (2nd edn, 1983), p.581.
27. See, for example, N. Ludmerer, 'Commentary' (1982) 8 *J Med Ethics* 92.
28. Lord Edmund-Davies, 'On dying and dying well—legal aspects' (1977) 70 *Proc R Soc Med* 73.
29. Lord Hailsham (1976) *The Listener*, 8 July, p.15.
30. See n.17 above.
31. N.24 above at p.289.
32. J. D. J. Havard, 'The legal threat to medicine' (1982) 284 *Brit Med J* 612.
33. J. D. J. Havard, 'Legal regulation of medical practice—decisions of life and death: A discussion paper' (1982) 75 *J Roy Soc Med* 351.
34. P. Devlin, *Easing the Passing* (1985) London: Bodley Head. See also the remarkable accusations made: *The Times* (1983) 11 July, p.2.
35. See n.28 above.
36. N.24 above, p.303.
37. N.24 above, p.303, J. Havard, 'Legislation is likely to cause more difficulties than it resolves' (1983) 9 *J Med Ethcs* 18.

CHAPTER THREE
Euthanasia

1. J. Glover, *Causing Death and Saving Lives* (reprinted 1986) Harmondsworth, Penguin, p.191.
2. J. Rachels 'Active and passive euthanasia' (1975) 292 *New Engl J Med* 78.
3. H. Kuhse, 'A modern myth. That letting die is not the intentional causation of death: Some reflections on the trial and acquittal of Dr Leonard Arthur' (1984) 1 *J Appl Philos* 21.
4. B. P. Gardner *et al*, 'Ventilation or dignified death for patients with high tetraplegia' (1985) 291 *Brit Med J* 1620. See also a similar tendency in the United States: S. E. Bedell and T. L. Delbanco, 'Choices about cardiopulmonary resuscitation in the hospital' (1984) 310 *New Engl J Med* 1089.
5. Lord Edmund-Davies, 'On dying and dying well' (1977) 70 *Proc R Soc Med* 73.
6. R. Nicholson, 'Should the patient be allowed to die?' (1975) 1 *J Med Ethics* 5.
7. (1957) 49 *Acta Apostolicae Sedis* 1027. The translation is mine and differs slightly from others I have read.
8. Sacred Congregation for the Doctrine of the Faith *Declaration on Euthanasia* (1980) Vatican: Polyglot Press. The article by J. J. McCartney, 'The development of the doctrine of ordinary and extraordinary means of

preserving life in Catholic moral theology before the Karen Quinlan case' (1981) 45 *Connecticut Med* 725 is very useful but, unfortunately, the source is not widely available. I believe that most readers would be surprised to learn how liberal the Catholic attitude is on this matter.

9. Well argued in C. Strong, 'Can fluids and electrolytes be "extraordinary" treatment?' (1981) 7 *J Med Ethics* 83. See also H. Kuhse, 'Extraordinary means and the sanctity of life' (1981) 7 *J Med Ethics* 74.

10. See Kuhse, n.9 above.

11. D. W. Meyers, *Medico-Legal Implications of Death and Dying* (1981) Rochester: The Lawyers Co-operative Publishing Co, at p.233 in discussion of *Satz v Perlmutter* 379 So 2d 359 (Fla, 1978).

12. W. Sweet, Quoted by I. M. Kennedy in 'The legal definition of death' (1973) 41 *Med-Leg J* 36.

13. J. E. Rhoads, 'The right to die and the chance to live' (1980) 6 *J Med Ethics* 53.

14. The comment is from the President's Commission for the Study of Ethical Problems in Medicine in their report *Deciding to Forego Life-sustaining Treatment* (1983). For a very useful review, see G. Dunea, 'When to stop treatment' (1983) 287 *Brit Med J* 1056.

15. J-O. Ottosson, quoted by J. Dawson, 'Easeful death' (1986) 293 *Brit Med J* 1187.

16. R. M. Veatch, *Death, Dying, and the Biological Revolution* (1976), p.42 quoted by P. D. G. Skegg in *Law, Ethics, and Medicine* (1984) Oxford: Clarendon Press.

17. This concept is elaborated by J. K. Mason and R. A. McCall Smith in *Law and Medical Ethics* (2nd edn, 1987), ch.15.

18. A. G. M. Campbell, 'The right to be allowed to die' (1983) 9 *J Med Ethics* 136.

19. R. Reiss, 'Moral and ethical issues in geriatric surgery' (1980) 6 *J Med Ethics* 71.

20. G. Williams, *Textbook of Criminal Law* (2nd edn, 1983) London: Sweet and Maxwell, p.279.

21. J. D. J. Havard, 'The influence of the law on clinical decisions affecting life and death' (1983) 23 *Med Sci Law* 157.

22. R. Ormrod, 'A lawyer looks at medical ethics' (1978) 46 *Med-Leg J* 18.

23. See Donaldson, M. R. in *Sidaway v Bethlem Royal Hospital Governors and others* [1984] 2 WLR 778.

24. *Barber v Superior Court of Los Angeles County and the People* 147 Cal App 3d 1006 (1983).

25. *In the matter of Claire C. Conroy* 464 A 2d 303 (NJ, 1983).

26. 486 A 2d 1209 (NJ, 1985).

27. For a review of these and other U.S. cases, see H. L. Hirsh and M. K. Cuneo, 'Who shall live, who shall die. Who decides?' (1986) 5 *Med Law* 111.

28. See A. Norberg *et al*, 'Ethical problems in feeding patients with advanced dementia' (1980) 281 *Brit Med J* 847 for a sensitive appraisal of the difficulties.

29. D. W. Meyers, *Medico-Legal Implications of Death and Dying* Rochester: The Lawyers Co-operative Publishing Co., Cum. Supp. (1984), p.84.

30. *The Sanctity of Life and the Criminal Law* (1958) London: Faber and Faber, p.280.
31. Parl Deb, HL, vol.169, 25 November, 1950.
32. Leading Article 'The King's peace?' (1986) *The Times*, 28 November, p.17.
33. *The Times*, 19 December 1986, p.7.
34. Lorber, n.5, ch.1, refused to accept active euthanasia in his paediatric practice but acknowledged that there was no real reason for so doing.
35. British Medical Association *The Problem of Euthanasia* (1971) London: BMA.
36. A. M. Capron, 'Legal and ethical problems in decisions for death' (1986) 14 *Law Med Hlth Care* 141.
37. J. Dawson, 'Easeful death' (1986) 293 *Brit Med J* 1187.
38. *The Sunday Times*, 30 November 1986, p.1.
39. N.20 above, p.580. See also R. Leng, 'Mercy killing and the CLRC' (1982) 132 *NLJ* 76.
40. *R v Byrne* [1960] 2 QB 396. This relatively strict interpretation has, admittedly, been markedly modified—*R v Seers* (1984) TLR, 5 May.
41. For discussion, see S. J. Morse, 'Undiminished confusion in diminished capacity' (1984) 75 *J Crim Law Criminol* 1; S. Dell, *Murder into Manslaughter* (1984). Oxford: University Press.
42. See, for example, *R v Johnson* (1971) 1 *Med Sci Law* 192 in which a father killed his mongol son by gassing. He was given a minimal sentence.

CHAPTER FOUR
Suicide
1. G. H. Gordon, *The Criminal Law of Scotland* (2nd edn, 1978) Edinburgh: W. Green, p.727 is surprisingly unhelpful on the subject—probably because of the near certainty that there is no criminality in suicide.
2. Schreiber, J. noted in *Conroy* 486 A 2d 1209 (NJ, 1985) that there was a difference between self-infliction or self-destruction and self-determination which was the basis for declining life-sustaining medical treatment. See also G. Williams, *The Sanctity of Life and the Criminal Law* (1958) London: Faber and Faber, p.245.
3. Lord Devlin, *Samples of Law Making* (1962) Oxford: University Press. See also I. Kennedy, 'The legal effect of requests by the terminally ill and aged not to receive further treatment from doctors' [1976] Crim LR 217 who discusses the matter within a broad range of problems.
4. P. D. G. Skegg, 'A justification for medical procedures performed without consent' (1974) 90 LQR 512 believed there was an overwhelming case for intervention by a doctor in any case where there was no reason to believe that the determination on self-destruction was fixed and unalterable.
5. *John F. Kennedy Memorial Hospital v Heston* 279 A 2d 670 (NJ, 1971) although this decision was reversed in *Conroy*, n.2 above.
6. This expression implies a sociological approach and, again, it is questioned whether one can commit legal suicide by omission. It is, however, hard to see how else such deaths could be classified and coroners' juries have returned verdicts of suicide on dead hunger-strikers. See Skegg, n.4 above.
7. An exhaustive review is given by G. Zellick in 'The forcible feeding of prisoners: An examination of the legality of enforced therapy' [1976] *Public Law* 153.

8. This was the basis of the early legal approach to force-feeding in the United Kingdom: *Leigh v Gladstone* (1909) 26 TLR 139—a case which has been widely criticised.

9. *In the matter of Von Holden v Chapman* (1982) 87 AD 2d 66.

10. *In re Joel Caulk* 480 A 2d 93 (NH, 1984).

11. See *In re Ramon Sanchez* 577 F Supp 7 (NY, 1983).

12. *Bouvia v The Superior Court of Los Angeles County* 179 Cal App 3d 1127.

13. The result would, therefore, depend very much on the conditions of the individual case. Damages were awarded in *Selfe v Ilford and District Hospital Management Committee* (1970) 114 SJ 935 but an appeal against a similar award was upheld in *Hyde v Tameside Area Health Authority* (1981) TLR 16 April.

14. G. Williams, *Textbook of Criminal Law* (2nd edn, 1983) London: Stevens, p.580. Williams says that a case of consent killing is occasionally reduced to a charge of assisting suicide.

15. J. F. Archbold, *Pleading, Evidence and Practice in Criminal Cases* (ed. Mitchels, 40th edn, 1979) London: Sweet and Maxwell.

16. M. P. Furmston, 'Is there a right to die?' (1981) 20 *Pol Surg* 7.

17. Note that this refers to a respirator which is used for the treatment of peripheral respiratory failure and is now very rare due to the virtual elimination of acute anterior poliomyelitis. The argument cannot be applied to the commonly used ventilator where respiratory failure is central in origin (see Chapter 5).

18. I. Kennedy, 'The legal effect of requests by the terminally ill and aged not to receive further treatment from doctors' [1976] Crim LR 217.

19. N.14 above, p.579.

20. *Attorney General v Able and others* (1983) TLR 29 April.

21. J. K. Mason and R. A. McCall Smith, *Law and Medcal Ethcs* (2nd edn, 1987) p.237.

CHAPTER FIVE
Brain Damage and Death

1. It would be reasonable to consider that the ventilator, in providing rhythmical respiration to the comatose patient, is, in fact, substituting for the respiratory centre in the brain. It is, however, easier to think in terms of it replacing pulmonary *function*.

2. W. Sweet. Quoted by I. M. Kennedy who also agrees that the intrinsic quality of life is the ability of the brain to support the body: 'The legal definition of death' (1973) 41 *Med-Leg J* 36.

3. Lord Scarman, 'Legal liability and medicine' (1981) 74 *J Roy Soc Med* 11.

4. P. Mollaret and M. Goulon, 'Le coma depassé' (1959) 101 *Rev Neurol* 3.

5. A. Mohandas and S. N. Chou, 'Brain death; a clinical and pathological study' (1971) 35 *J Neurosurg* 211.

6. H. K. Beecher (Chairman), 'A definition of irreversible coma' (1968) 205 *J Amer Med Ass* 337.

7. B. Jennett and F. Plum, 'Persistent vegetative state after brain damage' [1972] 1 *The Lancet* 734.

8. J. K. Mason, 'Medico-legal aspects of brain death' 1 *Int J Med Law* 205. See also A. Van Till-d'Aulnis de Bourouill, 'How dead can you be?' (1975) 15 *Med Sci Law* 133.

9. P. D. Skegg, 'Irreversibly comatosed individuals: alive or dead?' (1974) 33 *Cambridge LJ* 130.
10. G. Williams, 'Euthanasia' (1973) 41 *Med-Leg J* 14; Scarman, n.3 above.
11. Lord Edmund-Davies (1977), 'On dying and dying well' 70 *Proc R Soc Med* 73.
12. This follows from a long line of classic philosophical teaching, for example, Locke and Kant. The theory is currently being adapted and expanded. See, *inter alia*, J. Fletcher, 'Indications of humanhood: A tentative profile of man' (1972) 2 *Hastings Center Report*, No. 5; M. Tooley, *Abortion and Infanticide* (1983) Oxford: Clarendon Press; H. Kuhse and P. Singer, *Should the Baby Live?* (1985) Oxford: University Press.
13. H. Kuhse, 'Extraordinary means and the sanctity of life' (1981) 7 *J Med Ethics* 74.
14. I. M. Kennedy, 'Switching off life support machines: the legal implications' [1977] Crim LR 443.
15. G. S. Robertson, 'Dealing with the brain-damaged old—dignity before sanctity' (1982) 8 *J Med Ethics* 173.
16. E. Slater, 'Severely malformed children: Wanted—a new basic approach' [1973] 1 *Brit Med J* 285.
17. D. Coggan, 'On dying and dying well—moral and spiritual aspects' (1977) 70 *Proc R Soc Med* 75.
18. J. K. Mason and R. A. McCall Smith, *Law and Medical Ethics* (2nd edn, 1987), ch. 16. A good review of the problem is to be found in H. J. J. Leenen, 'The selection of patients in the event of a scarcity of medical facilities—an unavoidable dilemma' (1979) 1 *Int J. Med Law* 161. See also R. Gillon, 'Justice and allocation of medical resources' (1985) 291 *Brit Med J* 266.
19. *Re Quinlan* 355 A 2d 647 (NJ, 1976).
20. 1978 SLT (Notes) 60. See also A. A. Watson *et al*, 'Brain stem death: the Finlayson case' (1978) 23 *J Law Soc Scot* 433.
21. 'Diagnosis of brain death' [1976] 2 *Brit Med J* 1187.
22. 'Diagnosis of death' [1979] 1 *Brit Med J* 332.
23. But one or both of these tests is required in several countries including many of the States in America. The subject is discussed in detail by C. Pallis, *ABC of Brain Stem Death* (1983) London: BMA.
24. See, for example, articles of the type 'When does a beating heart die?' (1986) *The Sunday Times*, 7 December, p.1.
25. P. D. G. Skegg, 'The case for a statutory "definition of death"' (1976) 2 *J Med Ethics* 190; A. McCall Smith, 'Brain death: a case for legislation?' (1980) 25 *J Law Soc Scot* 113.
26. E.g. Human Tissue Act 1983 (NSW), s.33 or Human Tissue Act 1982 (Vict), s.41. Nevertheless, in the latter case, for example, the guidelines for diagnosis are those for the diagnosis of brain stem death.
27. A. Samuels, 'Death and the law—medico-legal problems' (1983) 23 *Med Sci Law* 183.
28. B. Jennett, 'Brain death 1981' (1981) 28 *Scott Med J* 191—elaborated by Pallis, n.23 above, pp.22-3.
29. I. Kennedy, *The Quality of Death* (1976) Illinois: Templegate, p.87, quoted by Lord Edmund-Davies (n.11 above).

30. N. 14 above.
31. G. Williams, n. 10 above.
32. G. Williams, 'Life of a child' (1981) *The Times*, 13 August, p. 7.
33. N. 30 above.
34. D. Brahams and M. Brahams, 'The Arthur case—a proposal for legislation' (1983) 9 *J Med Ethics* 12.
35. N. 20 above. The earlier case of *Re Potter* (1963) 31 *Med-Leg J* 195 scarcely provides a precedent.
36. N. 22 above.
37. *R* v *Malcherek, R* v *Steel* [1981] 2 All E R 422, CA.
38. J. J. Paris, 'Terminating treatment for newborns: a theological perspective' (1982) 10 *Law Med Hlth Care* 120. But it must be pointed out that this is a Jesuit view. One could pick out a Franciscan opinion: 'There is no right to death—on the contrary, there is a right to life' (quoted by S. Jacobson in 'The right to life' (1979) 19 *J Forens Sci Soc* 87).
39. See, for example, the Californian case of *People* v *Lyons* Alameda Co., Sup Ct, No 56072 (Calif, 1974) in which it was found that the victim of a shooting accident was legally dead before being used as a transplant donor.
40. 355 A 2d 647 (NJ, 1976).
41. K. Bai, 'Around the Karen Quinlan case: Interview with Judge R. Muir' (1979) 1 *Int J Med Law* 45.
42. N. 40 above, p. 663.
43. O. L. Wade, 'Research Ethical Committee' in A. S. Duncan *et al* (eds.) *Dictionary of Medical Ethics* (Revised, 1981) London: Darton, Longman and Todd, p. 371. See also P. J. Lewis, 'The drawbacks of research ethics committees' (1982) 8 *J Med Ethics* 61.
44. J. Goldstein, 'Medical care for the child at risk: on State supervention of parental autonomy' (1977) 86 *Yale L J* 645. I have seen only one recommendation for such an extension in the United Kingdom: A. Samuels, n. 27 above.
45. The issue in *Quinlan* was the right to refuse treatment. The victim was not brain dead and lived in a persistent vegetative state for over ten years after withdrawal from the ventilator.
46. *In re Storar* 438 NYS 2d 266 (NY, 1981) (consolidating *Eichner* v *Dillon*).
47. A concept involving 'donning the mental mantle' of an incompetent person so as to act on the same motives and considerations as would have moved the individual; see *Superintendent of Belchertown State School* v *Saikewicz* 370 NE 2d 417 (Mass, 1977).
48. L. J. Dunn, 'The *Eichner/Storar* decision: a year's perspective' (1982) 10 *Law Med Hlth Care* 117.
49. President's Commission for the Study of Ethical Problems in Medicine and Biomedical and Behavioral Research *Deciding to Forego Life-Sustaining Treatment* (1983) Washington DC: USGPO.
50. *Matter of Colyer* 660 P 2d 738 (Wash, 1983).
51. *Saikewicz*, n. 47 above. This was a treatment decision rather than a matter of brain death.
52. *John F. Kennedy Memorial Hospital* v *Bludworth* 452 So 2d 921 (Fla, 1984).
53. See, for example, A. S. Relman, 'The Saikewicz decision: Judges as physicians' (1978) 298 *New Engl J Med* 508; G. Dunea, 'When to stop treatment' (1983) 287 *Brit Med J* 1056.

54. E.g. California Durable Power of Attorney for Health Care Act, Cal Civ Code, s. 2430 *et seq.* Discussed by F. J. Collins and D. W. Meyers, 'Using a durable power of attorney for the authorization of withdrawal of medical care' [1984] *Estate Planning* 282.
55. E.g. California Natural Death Act 1976; Florida Life-Prolonging Procedures Act 1984.
56. M. Lappé, 'Dying while living: a critique of allowing-to-die legislation' (1978) 4 *J Med Ethics* 195.
57. Jacobson, n.38 above.
58. *Barber v Superior Court of Los Angeles County; Nejdl v same* (1983) 147 Cal App 3d 1006.
59. *Per* Crahan, J. Quoted by B. Towers in 'Public debate on issues of life and death' (1983) 9 *J Med Ethics* 113. There is an interesting association between these remarks and those of Lord Denning MR in *Lim Poh Choo v Camden and Islington Area Health Authority* [1979] 1 All ER 332, CA; both, although in different contexts, point to the importance of *admission* to the ventilator.
60. E.g. *Commonwealth v Golston* 366 NE 2d 744 (Mass. 1977); *In the matter of JN* 406 A 2d 1215 (DC Ct of App, 1979); *People v Lyons* 15 Crim L Rpt 2240, Cal Sup Ct (1974). The exception seems to be the rather old case of *People v Flores* Cal Sup Ct, County, 7246-C (1974).
61. No. 2831 (Richmond Va., L & Eq Court May 23, 1972). See also the test case *New York City Health and Hospitals Corporation v Sulsona*, 367 N Y S 2d 686 (Sup Ct Special Term, 1975).
62. For a full explanation, see D. W. Meyers, *Medico-Legal Implications of Death and Dying* (amended 1984) Rochester: The Lawyers Co-operative, ch.16.
63. Quoted by J. E. Cook and L. Hirsh, 'The legal implications of brain death' (1982) 1 *Med Law* 135. For a debate on the diagnosis see G. R. Gillett, 'Why let people die?' (1986) 12 *J Med Ethics* 83; J. M. Stanley, 'More fiddling with the definition of death' 13 *J Med Ethics* 21.

CHAPTER SIX
The Neonate

1. This is defined as the first twenty-eight days of life. To all intents, however, we are concerned with the first seventy-two hours which is the essential time for the *making* of neonatal decisions.
2. H. Kuhse and P. Singer, *Should the Baby Live?* (1985) Oxford: University Press, ch.5 is wholly concerned to show this.
3. The modern theory seems to have been developed at much the same time by J. Fletcher, 'Indications of humanhood: A tentative profile of man' (1972) 2 *Hastings Center Report*, No.5 and by M. Tooley, 'A defense of abortion and infanticide' in J. Feinberg (ed.) *The Problem of Abortion* (1973) Belmont: Wadsworth, p.51.
4. N.2 above, p.138.
5. This word has to be used because infanticide is strictly confined in English law to the killing of an infant by its mother.
6. D. Brahams, 'Putting Arthur's case in perspective' [1986] Crim LR 387.
7. E.g. Lord Scarman 'Legal liability and medicine' (1981) 74 *J Roy Soc Med* 11.

8. J(oseph) Fletcher, n.3 above.
9. J. Glover, *Causing Death and Saving Lives* (reprinted 1986) Harmondsworth: Penguin, p.138.
10. J(ohn) Fletcher, 'Abortion, euthanasia, and care of defective newborns' (1975) 292 *New Engl J Med* 75.
11. A very reasonable description is to be found in A. E. H. Emery, *Elements of Medical Genetics* (6th edn, 1983) Edinburgh: Churchill Livingstone.
12. R. Sherlock, 'Selective non-treatment of newborns' (1979) 5 *J Med Ethics* 139.
13. D. D. Matson, 'Surgical treatment of myelomeningocele' (1968) 42 *Pediatrics* 225.
14. J. Lorber, 'Ethical problems in the management of myelomeningocele' (1975) 10 *J R Coll Physns* 47.
15. J. Lorber and S. A.. Salfield, 'Result of selective treatment of spina bifida cystica' (1981) 56 *Arch Dis Childh* 822.
16. See 'Withholding treatment in infancy' (1981) 282 *Brit Med J* 925. Also A. G. M. Campbell and R. S. Duff, 'Deciding the care of severely malformed or dying infants' (1979) 5 *J Med Ethics* 65; R. S. Illingworth, 'The right to live and the right to die' (1981) 283 *Brit Med J* 612.
17. G. Williams, 'Down's syndrome and the duty to preserve life' (1981) 131 *NLJ* 1020.
18. D. Brahams, 'Acquittal of paediatrician charged after death of infant with Down syndrome' [1981] 2 *The Lancet* 1101. See also J. J. Paris and A. B. Fletcher, 'Infant Doe regulations and the absolute requirement to use nourishment and fluids for the dying infant' (1983) 11 *Law Med Hlth Care* 210.
19. Paris and Fletcher, n.18 above. D. Poole, 'Arthur's case (1) A comment' [1986] *Crim LR* 383.
20. (1981) *The Times*, 6 October, p.1.
21. Quoted from the transcript of the trial by D. Brahams and M. Brahams 'R v Arthur—is legislation appropriate?' (1981) 78 *Law Soc Gaz* 1342.
22. *In re B (A minor) (Wardship: Medical treatment)* [1981] 1 WLR 1421, CA.
23. Although Brahams (n.6 above) reported that, in fact, the infant died at the age of six years.
24. Per Dunn, L. J. [1981] 1 WLR at 1425.
25. *The Times* (1981) 6 November, p.1.
26. A. Usher, 'Correspondence' (1982) 284 *Brit Med J* 416.
27. J. K. Mason, 'Unresolved issues in Dr Arthur's case' (1981) *The Times*, 7 November, p.7. It is fair to say that Ian Kennedy does not support this view. See 'Reflections on the Arthur trial' (1982) 59 *New Society* No. 999, 7 January, p.13. But see, also, Brahams, n.6 above.
28. A fact which has made Williams appeal again for a relaxation of the mandatory sentence: 'Down's syndrome and the doctor's responsibility' (1981) 131 *NLJ* 1040.
29. See the large correspondence in (1981) 283 *Brit Med J* 1542; (1982) 284: pp.47-8, 415-16 in particular, perhaps, D. J. Gee and M. A. Green, at p.416. Also, J. Havard, 'Legislation is likely to create more difficulties than it resolves' (1983) 9 *J Med Ethics* 18; J. K. Mason, 'Expert evidence in the adversarial system of criminal justice' (1986) 26 *Med Sci Law* 8.

30. N. 18 above.
31. M. J. Gunn and J. C. Smith, 'Comments on comments' [1986] Crim LR 390.
32. R. Gillon, 'An introduction to philosophical medical ethics: the Arthur case' (1985) 290 *Brit Med J* 1117.
33. M. J. Gunn and J. C. Smith, '*Arthur's* case and the right to life of a Down's syndrome child' [1985] Crim LR 705.
34. G. Williams, 'Life of a child' (1981) *The Times*, 13 August, p.7.
35. Editorial Comment 'The right to live and the right to die' (1981) 283 *Brit Med J* 569.
36. E. F. Paul and J. Paul, 'Self ownership, abortion and infanticide' (1979) 5 *J Med Ethics* 133.
37. Brahams, see n. 18 above.
38. All the limitations on parental control which were set out in *Gillick* v *West Norfolk and Wisbech Area Health Authority and another* [1985] 3 WLR 830, HL depend upon the child's understanding of treatment options; they are, therefore, wholly inapplicable to the neonate.
39. Medical News (1981) 283 *Brit Med J* 567.
40. Gunn and Smith, n. 33 above.
41. Children Act 1975, s.85. For further comment, see Sherlock, n. 12 above.
42. A. J. Ayer, 'Why the Dr Arthur verdict is right' (1981) *The Times*, 6 November, p.14.
43. T. S. Ellis, 'Letting defective babies die: Who decides?' (1982) 7 *Amer J Law Med* 393.
44. Sherlock, n. 12 above.
45. J. M. Maciejczyk, 'Withholding treatment from defective infants: "Infant Doe" post mortem' (1983) 59 *Notre Dame LR* 224.
46. M. J. Garland, 'Care of the newborn: the decision not to treat' (1977) 1 *Perinat/Neonate* 14.
47. McKay v. *Essex Area Health Authority* [1982] 2 WLR 890.
48. B. M. Dickens, 'Withholding paediatric medical care' (1984) 62 *Canad Bar Rev* 196, discussing *Dawson*, n. 97 below.
49. Ellis, n. 43 above; Paris and Fletcher, n. 18 above.
50. See F. S. MacMillan, 'Birth defectve infants. A standard for non-treatment decisions' (1978) 30 *Stanford L Rev* 599.
51. N. 17 above.
52. Gunn and Smith, n. 31 above.
53. Re F; F v F (1986). Unreported, Sup Ct Victoria, 2 July.
54. See n. 17 above. Though the evidence is that compassion would be shown. The decision to charge Dr Arthur with murder is even less comprehensible in the light of the precedents.
55. N. 28 above.
56. N. 34 above.
57. Kennedy, n. 27 above.
58. J. M. Freeman, 'Is there a right to die—quickly?' (1972) 80 *J Pediat* 904. See also J. Harris, 'Ethical problems in the management of some severely handicapped children' (1981) 7 *J Med Ethics* 117.
59. H. Kuhse, 'A modern myth. That letting die is not the intentional causation of death: some reflections on the trial and acquittal of Dr Leonard

Arthur' (1984) 1 *J Appl Philos* 21 argues forcefully that there is no difference in law.

60. N.6 above.
61. Official Reports, March 1982. Written answers, cols 348-9.
62. N.21 above.
63. N.28 above.
64. Brahams, n.18 above.
65. See Brahams, n.21 above. There is case law to support the possibility (*R* v *Gibbins and Proctor* (1918) 13 Cr App Rep 134) but there seems to be no certainty on the point: A. E. Munir, 'Perinatal rights' (1984) 24 *Med Sci Law* 31.
66. Legal Correspondent 'Dr Leonard Arthur: his trial and its implications' (1981) 283 *Brit Med J* 1340. The same author's suggestion that defective neonates might be classed as 'monsters' and hence not 'reasonable creatures in being' who could not, therefore, be murdered seems unlikely to find general favour.
67. But it is widespread in the United States. See, for example, H. S. Shapiro, 'Medical treatment of defective newborns: an answer to the "Baby Doe" dilemma' (1983) 20 *Harvard J Legis* 137.
68. N.34 above.
69. *The Sunday Times* (1981) 9 April, p.3.
70. J. D. J. Havard, 'Legal regulation of medical practice—decisions of life and death: a discussion paper' (1982) 75 *J Roy Soc Med* 351.
71. Leading Article 'After the trial at Leicester' [1981] 2 *The Lancet* 1085.
72. A. Smith, 'The ethics of society rather than medical ethics' (1982) 8 *J Med Ethics* 120.
73. An interesting appraisal by a medical student is to be found in P. Ferguson, 'Paternalism versus autonomy: medical opinion and ethical questions in the treatment of defective neonates' (1983) 9 *J Med Ethics* 16. It is, of course, Kennedy's major criticism of modern medicine: see *The Unmasking of Medicine* (1981) London: George Allen and Unwin.
74. The reported surveys are often persuasive but tend to involve small numbers; it is often difficult to establish the degree of subjectivity involved. See B. Shepperdson, 'Abortion and euthanasia of Down's syndrome children—the parents' view' (1983) 9 *J Med Ethics* 152; M. Simms, 'Informed dissent: the views of some mothers of severely mentally handicapped young adults' (1986) 12 *J Med Ethics* 72.
75. N.35 above.
76. J. Lorber. Quoted by A. Ferriman, 'Doctor tells of the babies who are allowed to die' (1981) *The Times*, 13 August, p.1.
77. Editorial Comment 'Paediatricians and the law' (1981) 283 *Brit Med J* 1280.
78. Havard, n.29 above; n.70 above; J. D. J. Havard, 'The legal threat to medicine' (1982) 284 *Brit Med J* 612.
79. See, for example, R. B. Zachary, 'Correspondence' (1981) 283 *Brit Med J* 1463; or J. C. Murdoch at p.1464.
80. M. Blackwell, 'Correspondence' (1981) 283 *Brit Med J* 1463. See also Kuhse, n.59 above.
81. N.27 above.
82. N.29 above.

83. Havard, n.70 above.
84. Blackwell, n.80 above.
85. Editorial Comment 'Death without concealment' (1981) 283 *Brit Med J* 1629.
86. *Handbook of Medical Ethics* (1984) London: BMA, para. 10.21.
87. *The Scotsman* (1983) 13 May, p.10.
88. See, for example, Sherlock, n.12 above; Paris and Fletcher, n.18 above; Ellis, n.43 above.
89. An outstanding review of U.S. cases is to be found in L. Gostin, 'A moment in human development: legal protection, ethical standards and social policy on the selective non-treatment of handicapped neonates' (1985) 11 *Amer J Law Med* 31.
90. *Maine Medical Center v Houle* (1974) Maine, Cumberland Co Sup Ct No 74-145.
91. *In re McNulty* (1978) Mass., Probate Ct No. 1960 (the defect included congenital heart disease).
92. *Re Cicero* 421 NYS 2d 965 (1979).
93. *Custody of a Minor* 379 NE 2d 1053 (Mass, 1978).
94. *Weber v Stony Brook Hospital* 456 NE 2d 1186 (NY, 1983); US 104 S Ct 560 (1983).
95. *Guardianship of Phillip B* (1981) 139 Cal App 3d 407.
96. See n.89 above.
97. *Re Superintendent of Family and Child Service and Dawson* et al (1983) 145 DLR (3d) 610.
98. *Infant Doe v Bloomington Hospital* (1982) Ind., Monroe Co Cir Ct No GU 8204-004; US 104 S Ct 394 (1983).
99. *American Academy of Pediatrics v Heckler* 561 F Supp 395 (DCC, 1983).
100. *American Hospital Association v Heckler* 105 S Ct 3475 (1985).
101. See N. Lund, 'Infanticide, physicians and the law: the "Baby Doe" amendments to the Child Abuse Prevention and Treatment Act' (1985) 11 *Amer J Law Med* 1. See also Gostin, n.89 above.
102. See Brahams and Brahams, n.21above; Havard, n.29 above. For further discussion see J. K. Mason and R. A. McCall Smith, *Law and Medical Ethics* (2nd edn, 1987) London: Butterworths, p.113.
103. N.29 above.
104. V. Y. H. Yu et al, 'Prognosis for infants born at 23 to 28 weeks' gestation' (1986) 293 *Brit Med J* 1200.

CHAPTER SEVEN
Abortion

1. Other more unusual times have been suggested—e.g. the time after which the embryo cannot be maintained *in vitro* or at which cryopreservation is lethal. Such criteria are inconsistent as they depend upon changing technical abilities.
2. Infanticide is defined in England and Wales by the Infanticide Act 1938 under which it can *only* be committed by a mother in respect of her child under the age of twelve months; it does not carry a mandatory sentence. Deliberate killing of a neonate by any other person is murder or, in special circumstances, manslaughter. The Infanticide Act does not run to Scotland where the equivalent offence is known as child murder.
3. 93 S Ct 705 (1973).

4. George III, ch.58, 1803. To procure a miscarriage or abortion when quick with child was a capital offence; to do so before quickening was proved carried a lesser penalty—albeit running to transportation for up to fourteen years!

5. Witness the Declaration of Geneva. For a review of the relevant literature, see R. N. Wennberg, *Life in the Balance* (1985) Grand Rapids: Eerdmans.

6. See J. T. Noonan, 'An almost absolute value in history' in J. T. Noonan (ed.) *The Morality of Abortion* (1970) Harvard: University Press.

7. N.5 above, p.66.

8. In the sense that, for example, the contents of the bowel are 'external' to the body.

9. 'A surgeon' in K. Boyd *et al, Life before Birth* (1986) London: SPCK, pp.36-7.

10. The 1861 Act does not run to Scotland where the common law approach to abortion is similar, but not identical, to English law. There is little point in enlarging on Scots law in the present context.

11. G. Williams, *Textbook of Criminal Law* (2nd edn, 1983) London: Sweet and Maxwell, p.292.

12. [1939] 1 KB 687, [1938] 3 All ER 615.

13. It is still the foundation of therapeutic abortion in, say, Western Australia.

14. The quotations are from the All ER version at 618 and 619. There are minor differences in the Law Report.

15. See also *R v Newton and Stungo* [1958] Crim LR 469 and 600.

16. D. Baird, 'Induced abortion: Epidemiological aspects' (1975) 1 *J Med Ethics* 122.

17. J. M. Finnis, 'Three schemes of regulation' in Noonan, n.6 above, put the annual figure at anything between 10000 and 100000.

18. The 1967 Act does not apply to Northern Ireland.

19. P. T. O'Neill and I. Watson, 'The father and the unborn child' (1975) 38 *MLR* 174.

20. *Paton v United Kingdom* (1980) 3 EHRR 408. A rather desperate attempt has been made to show that a father could, at least under Scots law, apply for and obtain guardianship of his developing child but it is difficult to believe that this would be accepted in view of the European decision; see D. M. Yorke, 'The personality of the unborn child' (1979) SLT 158. See also *C v S* (1987) TLR, 24 an 25 February, discussed in detail in Chapter 9.

21. *McKay v The Essex Area Health Authority* [1982] 2 WLR 890.

22. J. D. J. Havard, 'Therapeutic abortion' [1958] Crim LR 600.

23. *Emeh v Kensington and Chelsea and Westminster Area Health Authority* [1984] 3 All ER 1044, CA.

24. In *McKay*, n.21 above.

25. *Roe v Wade* 93 S Ct 705 (1973); *Doe v Bolton* 93 S Ct 739 (1973).

26. *American College of Obstetricians and Gynecologists, Pennsylvania Section and others v Thornburgh and others* 106 S Ct 2169 (1986).

27. *Harris v McRae* 100 S Ct 2671 (1980).

28. N.12 above.

29. *R v Davidson* [1969] VR 667; *R v Wald and others* (1971) 3 DCR (NSW) 25.

30. Although the unreported case of *Kambomogou v Crown St Women's Hospital* (1980) NSW Sup Ct suggests its legality (see P. Hersch, 'Tort liability for "wrongful life"' (1983) 6 U N S W L J 133).

31. Leading Article 'No case for an abortion Bill' [1979] 2 *Brit Med J* 230.
32. 'A general practitioner' in Boyd *et al*, n.9 above, p.40.
33. *R v Smith (John)* [1973] 1 WLR 1510.
34. N.15 above.
35. N.29 above.
36. Institute of Medical Ethics (1988) Bull. no 36, p.15.
37. J. Glover, *Causing Death and Saving Lives* (Reprinted 1986) Harmondsworth: Penguin, p.142.
38. T. Kushner, 'Having a life versus being alive' (1984) 10 *J Med Ethics* 5.
39. In O'Neill and Watson, n.19 above.
40. S. McLean and G. Maher, *Medicine, Morals and the Law* (1983) Aldershot: Gower, p.26.
41. J. Benschof, 'Reasserting women's rights' (1985) 17 *Fam Plan Perspect* 162.
42. J. T. Thomson, 'A defence of abortion' in P. Singer (ed.) (1986) *Applied Ethics*, Oxford: University Press, ch.4.
43. N.40 above, p.30.
44. N.3 above.
45. *Jefferson v Griffin Spalding County Hospital Authority* 274 SE 2d 457 (Ga, 1981).
46. *Taft v Taft* 446 NE 2d 395 (Mass, 1983).
47. D C. Bross and A. Meredyth, 'Neglect of the unborn child: an analysis based on law in the United States' (1979) 3 *Child Abuse Neg* 643. It is understood, however, that the prosecution of a Californian mother for contributing to the death of her fetus by drug-taking during pregnancy ((1986) *Guardian*, 2 October, p.8) was dismissed on the grounds that there was no case to answer.
48. *D (a minor) v Berkshire CC* [1987] 1 All ER 20; *Superintendent of Family and Child Service and McDonald* (1982) 135 DLR (3d) 330; *Re Children's Aid Society of Kenora and JL* (1982) 134 DLR (3d) 249.
49. E. W. Keyserlingk, 'A right of the unborn child to pre-natal care—the civil law perspective' (1982) 13 *Rev de Droit* 49.
50. N.40 above, p.31. See also Glover, n.37 above, p.146.
51. Church Assembly Board of Responsibility of the Church of England *Abortion: An Ethical Discussion* (1965) London: Church Information Office.
52. McKay, n 21 above.
53. P. Ramsey, 'Reference points in deciding about abortion' in J. T. Noonan, n.6 above.
54. Lord Wells-Pestell, 355 HL Official Report (5th series), col 776 (12 December 1974).
55. See the discussion in V. Tunkel, 'Abortion: how early, how late, and how legal?' [1979] 2 *Brit Med J* 253.
56. G. Wright, 'The legality of abortion by prostaglandin' [1984] Crim LR 347; V. Tunkel, 'Late abortions and the crime of child destruction': (1) A reply' [1985] Crim LR 133. It is to be noted that Tunkel has had a radical change of opinion since 1979. See now, *C v S*, n.20 above.
57. *Colautti v Franklin* 439 US 379 (1979).

58. Lane, Mrs Justice (Chrmn) Report of the Committee on the Working of the Abortion Act (1974) Cmnd 5579, London: HMSO, para 278.
59. M. A Somerville, 'Reflections on Canadian abortion law: evacuation and destruction—two separate issues' (1981) 31 U Toronto LJ 1. A similar position has been adopted in the United Kingdom: P. M. Dunn and G. M. Stirrat, 'Capable of being born alive?' [1984] 1 The Lancet 553.
60. V. Y. H. Yu et al, 'Prognosis for infants born at 23 to 28 weeks' gestation' (1986) 293 Brit Med J 1200.
61. B. Towers, 'The trials of Dr Waddill' (1979) 5 J Med Ethics 205. See also the rather similar case resulting in acquittal Commonwealth v Edelin 359 NE 2d 4 (Mass, 1976).
62. Inquest on Infant Campbell, Stoke on Trent, 19 October 1983.
63. R v Hamilton (1983) The Times, 16 September, p. 1.
64. K. McK. Norrie, 'Abortion in Great Britain: one Act, two laws' [1985] Crim LR 475.
65. (1983) The Times, 11 May, p. 1.
66. I. J. Keown, '"Miscarriage": a medico-legal analysis' [1984] Crim LR 604.
67. N. 4 above.
68. See the discussion of the correspondence in The Times (April 1983) in 'The post-coital pill: lawful or not?' (1983) 287 Brit Med J 64.
69. N. 58 above, para 92.
70. Abortion Act 1967, s. 5(2).

CHAPTER EIGHT
Embryocide

1. Department of Health, Education and Welfare: Ethics Advisory Board (1979) Report and Conclusions, 4 May.
2. Report of the Committee of Inquiry into Human Fertilisation and Embryology (M. Warnock, Chairman) (1984), Cmnd 9314.
3. B. Braine. Official Reports, HC, 23 November 1984, Col 540; J. Knight, Col 565.
4. First Report of the Voluntary Licensing Authority for Human in vitro Fertilisation and Embryology (1986), p. 8. The term has also been adopted by other bodies—e.g. the Ethics Committee of the American Fertility Society (1986) 46 Fertil Steril, Supp 1.
5. L. Walters, quoted by B. J. Culliton and W. K. Waterfall in 'Flowering of American bioethics' [1978] 2 Brit Med J 1270.
6. N. 2 above, p. 64.
7. Unborn Children (Protection) Bills 1985, 1986.
8. M. M. Quigley and L. B. Andrews, 'Human in vitro fertilization and the law' (1984) 42 Fertil Steril 348.
9. Infertility (Medical Procedures) Act 1984.
10. Institute of Medical Ethics, Bull 19, October 1986, p. 14.
11. Editorial Comment 'Common sense and contraception' (1983) The Times, 10 May, p. 13.
12. The point is made very clearly in K. Boyd et al, Life Before Birth (1986) London: SPCK, p. 116 et seq.
13. See Editorial Comment 'Values from the Vatican' (1987) The Times, 11 March, p. 13 and also p. 3.

14. T. Iglesias, 'In vitro fertilisation: The major issues' (1984) 10 J Med Ethics 32.

15. G. R. Dunstan, 'The moral status of the human embryo: A tradition recalled' (1984) 10 J Med Ethics 38.

16. N.12 above, p.146.

17. M. Warnock, A Question of Life (1985) Oxford: Blackwell, p.xiii.

18. P. Steptoe, 'The role of in vitro fertilization in the treatment of infertility: Ethical and legal problems' (1986) 26 Med Sci Law 82.

19. A particularly poignant example occurred in 1987. See I. Craft, 'When a code catches out the childless' (1987) The Times, 24 September, p.16.

20. In the seminal British case R v Dudley and Stephens (1884) 14 QBD 273, the court concluded that inactivity was the correct solution—which is unhelpful.

21. C. De Garis, H. Kuhse, P. Singer and V. Y. H. Yu, 'Attitudes of Australian neonatal paediatricians to the treatment of extremely preterm infants' (1987) 23 Aust Paediatr J 223.

22. McKay v The Essex Area Health Authority [1982] 2 WLR 890 at 902.

23. Second Report of the Voluntary Licensing Authority, 1987, p.12.

24. I. Craft et al, 'The fertility debate and the media' (1987) 295 Brit Med J 1134.

25. Craft, n.19 above.

CHAPTER NINE
An Overview

1. J. Harvard, 'Legislation is likely to create more difficulties than it resolves' (1983) 9 J Med Ethics 18; A. Smith, 'The ethics of society rather than medical ethics' (1982) 8 J Med Ethics 120.

2. Discussed by R. Gillon, 'To what do we have moral obligations and why? II' (1985) 290 Brit Med J 1734.

3. J. Lachs, 'Humane treatment and the treatment of humans' (1976) 294 New Engl J Med 838.

4. M. Tooley, 'A defense of abortion and infanticide' in J. Feinberg, The Problem of Abortion (1973) Belmont: Wadsworth, p.51.

5. A. G. M. Campbell, 'The right to be allowed to die' (1983) 9 J Med Ethics 136.

6. R. Klein, 'Rationing health care' (1984) 289 Brit Med J 143.

7. I. Kennedy, The Unmasking of Medicine (1981) London: George Allen & Unwin.

8. Quoted in R. G. Twycross, 'Euthanasia—a physician's viewpoint' (1982) 8 J Med Ethics 86.

9. G. Hughes, 'Commentary' (1981) 7 J Med Ethics 79. The debate with H. Kuhse, 'Extraordinary means and the sanctity of life' (1981) 7 J Med Ethics 74 provides a most thought-provoking expression of the subject.

10. G. Dunea, 'When to stop treatment' (1983) 287 Brit Med J 1056.

11. M. Siegler and A. J. Weisbard, 'Against the emerging stream' (1985) 145 Arch Intern Med 129.

12. For a review of the hospice system, see C. Saunders, 'Hospices' in A. S. Duncan et al. (eds.), Dictionary of Medical Ethics (Revised, 1981) London: Darton, Longman and Todd.

13. See, for example, P. J. F. Baskett, 'The ethics of resuscitation' (1986) 293 *Brit Med J* 189; R. I. S. Bayliss, 'Thou shalt not strive officiously' (1982) 285 *Brit Med J* 1373; or, in the United States, A. S. Relman, 'The Saikewicz decision: Judges as physicians' (1978) 298 *New Engl J Med* 508.

14. Twycross, n.8 above.

15. See, especially, J. Rachels, 'Active and passive euthanasia' (1975) 292 *New Engl J Med* 78. And, now, *The End of Life: Euthanasia and Morality* (1986) Oxford: University Press.

16. Law Reform Commission of Canada, *Criteria for the Determination of Death* Rep. no.15, 1981.

17. Human Tissue Act 1982, s.41 (Victoria); Human Tissue Act 1983, s.33 (NSW).

18. P. D. G. Skegg, *Law, Ethics, and Medicine* (1984) Oxford: Clarendon Press, p.210 discusses this at length and concludes that medical opinion is changing in that direction. See also the interesting debate J. M. Stanley, 'More fiddling with the definition of death?' (1987) 13 *J Med Ethics* 21 with reply by G. Gillett, 'Fiddling and clarity' (1987) 13 *J Med Ethics* 23.

19. G. S. Robertson (1984) *The Scotsman*, 2 October, p.9.

20. *In re Hier* 464 NE 2d 959 (Mass, 1984) (withdrawal of treatment allowed); *Brophy v New England Sinai Hospital Inc.* No. 85 E0009-GI, Probate Court (Mass, 1985) (withdrawal disallowed). Discussed by M. Swartz, 'The patient who refuses medical treatment: A dilemma for hospitals and physicians' (1985) 11 *Amer J Law Med* 147.

21. *Superintendent of Belchertown State School v Saikewicz* 370 NE 2d 417 (Mass, 1978).

22. *John F. Kennedy Memorial Hospital Inc v Bludworth* 452 So 2d 921 (Fla, 1984).

23. See, for example, the attempt in S. H. Wanzer *et al.*, 'The physician's responsibility towards hopelessly ill patients' (1984) 310 *New Engl J Med* 955.

24. [1957] Crim LR 365.

25. Catholic Bishops' Joint Committee on Bio-ethical Issues (England, Ireland, Scotland, Wales), *Care of the Handicapped Newborn* (1986) London: Catholic Media Office, para 5.3.

26. *The Sunday Times*, 11 May, 1986, p.3; *The Times*, 2 February, 1987, p.3.

27. Quoted by H. Kuhse, 'A modern myth. That letting die is not the intentional causation of death' (1984) 1 *J Appl Philos* 21.

28. M. J. Gunn and J. C. Smith, '*Arthur's* case and the right to life of a Down's syndrome child' [1985] Crim LR 705.

29. Editorial Comment, 'The right to live and the right to die' (1981) 283 *Brit Med J* 569.

30. Law Reform Commission of Canada (1982) Working paper no.28, quoted by Z. Lipman in 'The criminal liability of medical practitioners for withholding treatment from severely defective newborn infants' (1986) 60 *ALJ* 286.

31. J. K. Mason and R. A. McCall Smith, *Law and Medical Ethics* (2nd edn, 1987) London: Butterworths, p.115. The organisation 'Prospect' have lobbied Parliament with a Limitation of Treatment Bill—C. Gillespie (1983) 9 *J Med Ethics* 231.

32. G. P. Smith, 'Defective newborns and government intermeddling' (1985) 25 *Med Sci Law* 44.
33. J. K. Mason and D. W. Meyers, 'Parental choice and selective non-treatment of deformed newborns: A view from mid-Atlantic' (1986) 12 *J Med Ethics* 67.
34. L. Gostin, 'A moment in human development: Legal protection, ethical standards and social policy on the selective non-treatment of handicapped neonates' (1985) 11 *Amer J Law Med* 31.
35. Department of Health, Education and Welfare Ethics Advisory Board, *HEW Support of Research Involving Human In Vitro Fertilization and Embryo Transfer* 4 May, 1979.
36. N.27 above.
37. J. Kekef, 'Moral intuition' (1986) 23 *Amer Philosoph Quart* 83.
38. P. Tizard and T. L. Chambers, 'Human embryos' (1984) *The Times*, 1 June, p.13.
39. P. Ramsey, 'Abortion' (1973) 37 *Thomist* 174 quoted by J. Fletcher, 'Abortion, euthanasia and care of defective newborns' (1975) 292 *New Engl J Med* 75.
40. For discussion see J. Glover, *Causing Death and Saving Lives* (Reprinted 1986) Harmondsworth: Penguin Books, pp.140 et seq.
41. J. Connell, 'Death-wish prayers fuel abortion row' (1986) *The Sunday Times*, 15 June, p.12. See also J. D. Forrest and S. K. Henshaw, 'The harassment of US abortion providers' (1987) 19 *Fam Plan Perspect* 9.
42. B. Towers, 'The trials of Dr Waddill' (1979) 5 *J Med Ethics* 205.
43. *Gillick v West Norfolk and Wisbech Area Health Authority* [1983] 3 WLR 859, QBD; [1985] 2 WLR 413, CA; [1985] 3 WLR 830, HL.
44. Abortion Act 1967, s.5(1) in England and Wales; *Roe v Wade* 93 S Ct 705 (1973) in the United States.
45. Infant Life (Preservation) Act 1929. The ill-fated Infant Life (Preservation) Bill 1987 sought to clear up the uncertainties in the wording of this Act —Institute of Medical Ethics, Bull no.23, February 1987, p.4.
46. Births and Deaths Registration Act 1953, s.4; Registration of Births, Deaths and Marriages (Scotland) Act 1965, s.56.
47. The full WHO definition is given by P. R. Norris, 'Time, chance and the unborn child' (1987) *The Times*, 2 March, p.13.
48. *C v S* (1987) TLR, 24 February, QBD; 25 February, CA. For discussion, see C. Dyer, 'Father fails in attempt to stop girlfriend's abortion' (1987) 294 *Brit Med J* 631.
49. *The Times*, 1 June 1984, p.3; 3 August 1985, p.2. See also IME *Bulletin*, n.45 above. But the limit of eighteen weeks proposed in the Abortion (Amendment) Bill 1987 must, surely, be unreasonably low.
50. Abortion Act 1967, s.4.
51. P. Ramsey, 'Reference points in deciding about abortion' in J. T. Noonan (ed.), *The Morality of Abortion* (1970) Harvard: University Press.
52. D. Brahams, 'Putting *Arthur's* case in perspective' [1986] Crim LR 387.
53. N.44 above.
54. C. S. Rush, 'Genetic screening, eugenic abortion and *Roe v Wade*: How viable is *Roe's* viability standard?' (1983) 50 *Brooklyn L Rev* 113.

55. I foresee the need also for a subsection along the lines: 'Such a termination must still be subject to the mother's consent and, in the event of a refusal in good faith, no action in tort will be available to the child against its mother'.

56. *McKay v Essex Area Health Authority* [1982] 2 WLR 890.

57. Actions for wrongful life have succeeded in the United States: *Turpin v Sortini* 182 Cal Rptr 337 (1982); *Harbeson v Parke-Davis Inc* 656 P 2d 483 (Wash, 1983).

58. P. M. Dunn and G. M. Stirrat, 'Capable of being born alive?' [1984] 1 *The Lancet* 553.

59. See E. Alberman *et al.* 'Congenital abnormalities in legal abortions at 20 weeks' gestation or later' [1984] 1 *The Lancet* 1226; for review see P. Bromwich, 'Late abortion' (1987) 294 *Brit Med J* 527.

60. D. Callahan, 'How technology is reframing the abortion debate' (1986) 16 *Hastings Center Report* (1) 33.

61. J. Thynne, 'Oxford prays for its unborn child' (1987) *The Sunday Times*, 1 March, p. 1.

62. Editorial Comment, 'Values from the Vatican' (1987) *The Times*, 11 March, p. 13.

63. For a spirited expression of opposition to legalised abortion, see the view from West Germany: W. Esser, 'Can abortion be legally justified?' (1984) 3 *Med Law* 205.

64. In Towers, n. 42 above.

Index

TABLE OF CASES